# Aromaflexology

Combining essential oils and foot reflexes for good health

Shirley Price

Riverhead Publishing, Stratford-upon-Avon, Warwickshire, England
www.riverhead.co.uk

AROMAFLEXOLOGY

Combining essential oils and foot reflexes for good health

*Shirley Price*

*This edition first published 2018*
*© 2018 Shirley Price*
*© 2018 Riverhead Publishing*

*First Edition 2018*
*Reprinted with minor corrections 2019*

*British Library Cataloguing–in–Publication Data.*
*A catalogue record for this book is available from the British Library.*

*ISBN 978-1-874353-16-4*
*Set in Baskerville, 9½ on 12*
*Printed in England*
*Illustrations: Len Price*
*MMXVIII*

# Contents

# Foreword

When Shirley first asked me to write a foreword for this new book on Aromaflexology I was honored. Shirley Price is a treasured Aromatherapist and Reflexologist who has been sharing her knowledge and providing resources for professional complementary healthcare practitioners for decades. She has been my mentor and friend for many years and our personal and professional relationship has greatly enriched my life.

I had the privilege of studying distillation with Shirley and Len Price in France in 2004 where she gave our group an introduction to Aromaflexology (formerly Swiss Reflex Therapy). I invited them to bring their aromatherapy courses to the United States the following year, including Shirley's Aromaflexology class. The students were amazed as Shirley shared the results of many case studies with the class; especially the case study involving "Frank" and his remarkable recovery. At the conclusion of the class, Shirley approached me about teaching for her daughter's school (Penny Price Aromatherapy Academy). I later opened a satellite school in Chicago to teach the diploma program as well as Shirley's Aromaflexology certification class.

Aromaflexology provides the aromatherapist with much needed tools to "assess" their clients and provide a hands-on treatment using essential oils. In addition, it goes a step further, as the client (or the caregiver) receives instruction for daily home care which expedites the healing process. This is a win-win for the practitioner as most clients know what to expect when seeing most complementary providers, but are still in the dark about what an authentic aromatherapist does. Aromaflexology gives both practitioners and clients a tool that provides results. The specific dialogue between therapist and client yields far more information for the practitioner than filling in a client intake form/record sheet. This helps the therapist to select the most beneficial oils and to individualize the cream and application. I have also found that this results in a warmer relationship between client and therapist. In reflexology, the client is dependent on successive treatments from the therapist and can begin to react against the cost and the control by another. With Aromaflexology, the clients are more proactive in their own healthcare – they like to be in charge of their health and well-being and tend to return whenever the need arises.

This book fully explains the history and use of Aromaflexology. Shirley further explains the basis of Aromaflexology, the position of the reflex points and "hand-holds" as tools to assess the client's health, plus the hands-on application and instruction for the client or caregiver. She also discusses the "affirmative" dialogue to have with the client during the assessment and how it yields more information for the therapist. The book contains case studies, complete with protocols for care and the essential oils selected. There is a chapter dedicated to essential oil selection for a number of conditions by body system.

The book doesn't stop there. It also provides instruction for a shoulder massage to help reduce stress in your client. Stress is the underlying cause of dis-ease 70% of the time. This massage is a beneficial addition to enhance the therapy session. The book provides clear instruction and diagrams, which have been beautifully and clearly drawn by Len. Additionally, there is a section on suitable and safe Aromaflexology for babies. I have used it successfully with babies to ease constipation.

This long-awaited book is sure to enhance both your practice and the well-being of your clients. Kudos to Shirley for developing this wonderful technique and sharing it with the community at large. I am, as ever, grateful to Shirley (and Len) for their wonderful contributions to our aromatic community, their friendship, and love.

Lora Cantele, RA APAIA Certified Aromaflexologist

# Introduction –
# from Reflexology to Aromaflexology

In 1971 I qualified in reflexology with Doreen Bayley, a well known reflexologist who had studied with Dr William Fitzgerald and Eunice Ingham and was the first to open a school of reflexology in the UK.

Doreen Bayley was in her 70s when I went on her course and I have to say that in my opinion the classes were far too big to be able to teach a practical subject (50-60 people); nevertheless, I was smitten and decided to introduce the therapy to our health and beauty salon. On my return home, when explaining the art to my husband, he was very sceptical – indeed, he thought I had gone mad! It wasn't until I found his reactive lung reflexes (he is asthmatic), that he was amazed – and believed.

After studying reflexology, I attended three aromatherapy courses in London (Eve Taylor, Elizabeth Jones and William Arnould-Taylor). Again, the classes were far too big for practical learning, but one of the courses used the reflex points to help "diagnose" (I prefer the word "assess") the health of the client, which was interesting.

I was already qualified in body massage and have to admit that I found the movement involved in massage much more pleasurable than simple static pressure on reflex points. (I am one of those people who cannot talk without waving my hands and arms around!) Nevertheless, if reflexology was what my clients needed – that's what they were given!

Then – in 1987, we went to stay with friends in Switzerland – and the therapy Aromaflexology, founded on combining aromatherapy and reflexology, was evolved!

But first, let us look more closely at Reflexology.

## Reflexology

Reflexology is an ancient method of stimulating the body's healing forces, based on the belief that bodily organs are reflected in the feet through reflex points and that by applying pressure with the tip of the thumb on different parts of the feet a person's state of health and general well-being could be improved. It is a subject in its own right and learning the diagnostic techniques in aromaflexology does not qualify students and practitioners of the latter to give reflexology treatments, or to call themselves reflexologists.

The reflex points used in a reflexology treatment can be used to great advantage to assess the state of a person's health before carrying out a treatment such as aromatherapy, aromaflexology or body massage. The thumbs (and occasionally the fingers) are used on the reflex points which are found in the feet and hands (the tongue and ears also have reflex points which represent the bodily organs, but these are less commonly used). The reflex points on the feet are not only the most responsive, but are also the easiest on which to explain their relationship to the parts of the body being treated.

As each reflex area represents a specific part of the body, the subtle energy path linking the reflexes and the bodily organs enables reflexologists to treat the body simply by using pressure of varying depths on those reflexes. These cannot be seen by the human eye or on an X-ray or scan – they are subtle energies which make themselves felt when there is a health imbalance in the organ each represents.

How often have you said something and your spouse (or partner) was thinking exactly the same thing at exactly the same time? Telepathy, a way of communicating information from one person to another without using the five senses, is possible through subtle energy.

Basic energy (or Life Force) is found in every living thing, and human beings have an added dimension – that of intelligence, which gives us the ability to use and direct these energies in a way which can enhance our lives – or destroy them, as can happen with a negative thinking person. In both reflexology and aromaflexology, the therapist's aim is to facilitate the balancing of this energy. Through the feet or hands, a practitioner can help to identify energy blockages causing health concerns in a person's body, and by treating the reflex points and/or reflex areas, help that person to regain the natural balance needed to have a healthy body.

Conventional medicine often aims to make a person better by treating the symptoms of an illness – though unfortunately, rarely targets the cause. It has the added disadvantage of possible side effects given by tablets prescribed; tablets given for these side-effects can produce further, different, side-effects, which, in my mother's case, ended up with her having to take 22 tablets a day. Reflexology, aromaflexology and therapy using essential oils not only are devoid of side-effects and can help a person feel better (due to the removal of symptoms), but can also get to the cause of the illness, creating a whole new sense of wellness.

## Origins of Reflexology

No one culture can claim to have discovered reflexology, as foot massage has been used by people all over the world since the beginning of time (Issel 1990). It is also clear from historical records that the relationship between the feet and the internal organs of the body was recognised by civilisations way back in history.

As long ago as the Egyptian dynasty, treatment on the feet was common, in fact the oldest documentation of the use of reflexology is found in Egypt (Riley 1959); many of the wall drawings depict a person with their hands on another person's foot – unmistakeably representing a reflexology treatment (although it was not known by that name). Hieroglyphics above one of these murals have been translated, the patient saying "Do not let it be painful" and the therapist replying "I shall act so you praise me" (Adamson & Harris 1995). Ancient Egyptian doctors were the first to study the human body scientifically – they studied the structure of the brain and knew that the pulse was in some way connected with the heart (Issel p. 5). Not much is known of the development of reflexology after that, though ancient American Indians have practised the art for hundreds of years.

Dr. William Fitzgerald (1872-1942), an American ear, nose and throat specialist, is considered to be the father of reflexology as it is known today. He is credited with advancing and developing the initial popular practice of reflexology in our contemporary Western society (Scott Byrne 2012), discovering that pressure applied to certain points on the body could relieve pain and improve the functions of certain organs of the body. Having created the notion of zone therapy in 1909, Fitzgerald went on to develop a system of zones running from the top of the head to the tips of the toes and hands, and together with his colleague, Edwin Bowers, published his book "Zone Therapy" (1917), the name by which reflexology was known until the early 1960's.

"Because reflexology is linked with zone therapy, the reflex points on the feet are found in the same zones of the body, which run in straight lines from head to foot, both in the body and in the feet. There is no crossing over from one side of the body to the other – reflexes are all found in direct zone lines.

The reflexes which give discomfort when pressure is applied during an assessment indicate which organs require treatment."

Although fellow doctors did not express much interest in this book, one, Dr Joseph Shelby Riley, was intrigued by it. Fitzgerald shared information with Riley, who added eight horizontal divisions to Fitzgerald's longitudinal zones and made the first detailed diagrams of the reflex points located in the feet (O'Neil 2015). Riley taught the technique to his wife Elizabeth and also to his massage therapist, Eunice Ingham (1897-1974).

Eunice Ingham adapted Dr Riley's technique to her own liking, taking her form of the therapy to the non-medical public across the length and breadth of the United States, often facing harassment from the medical profession (Scott Byrne). According to Adamson and Harris, Eunice Ingham was the "true matriarch of zone therapy"; developing it and (very importantly) changing the name to reflexology – relating each sensitive spot on the feet to the organs of the body (Byers D 2001).

Eunice Ingham's nephew, Dwight Byers, inherited his aunt's organisation and continued where she left off after her death in 1974, setting up training centres in the U.S.A. with similar standards to the Bayly school. Doreen Bayly, who was taught by Eunice Ingham, brought her method to the UK in 1966/7, opening a school to teach reflexology (Byrne 2012). Her course was originally one weekend of practical training, after which each participant was issued a certificate. The course was later increased to two weekends (which I myself attended in London) to allow the students to practise between visits, making the awarding of a certificate a little more meaningful, although the certificates were given at the end of the course without an assessment or examination (students numbered 50-60 per class). Her book, "Reflexology – a Way to Better Health", was published in 1998 and is highly regarded. When Doreen Bayly died in 1976, the Bayly school was taken over by Nicola Hall who continued training the students along similar lines to Doreen Bayly.

In the UK a retired nurse, Gladys Evans, also worked on the feet from about the 1960s, with a combination of zone therapy and pressure points. She taught that too much pressure would tense the muscles in the client's body, which would impede the blood supply, thus leading to a build-up of toxins. The infliction of pain could also lead to further stress rather than the relaxation necessary to promote healing. (I became of the same mind as Gladys after having a reflexology treatment in Sweden by the proprietor of the school for which I was teaching aromatherapy. She had learned reflexology at a Swedish reflexology school and used her knuckles and a pencil (yes!) for the pressures. The pain was so excruciating that I had to recite poetry out loud to take my mind off the pain.

Gladys Evans exchanged her knowledge with various interested clients, friends and other practitioners of various reflexology methods, among whom were Doreen Bayly and Renée Tanner.

Today several versions of reflexology techniques exist, including the original Ingham method, the Bayly method, and the Tanner method, as well as more modern versions such as Vertical reflex therapy (Scott Byrne 2012).

The body has a remarkable capacity to regenerate itself, as is seen when a small cut or wound heals itself without outside help. The treatment of reflexes is a simple technique which can enable the regeneration of healthy cells to take place more quickly – and there are no detrimental side effects if correctly and sensitively administered.

Sir Henry Head, (1861 – 1940) was a neurologist who conducted pioneering work into the somatosensory system and sensory nerves in London. When in 1893, he published his discovery regarding the connection between spinal segments, skin sensitivity and internal organs, he wrote "the bladder can be excited into action by stimulating the soles of the feet" He discovered that these areas were connected through nerves to a diseased organ. (Scott Byrne 2012). After years of clinical research, Head established what became known as 'Heads Zones' or 'Zones of Hyperalgesia' (O'Neil 2015).

In the late 1890's and early 1900's, the Germans were developing massage techniques which became known as 'reflex massage' and it is believed they were the first to apply massage to 'reflex zones'.

But now – read on, to learn how I further developed the art of what began as zone therapy, then reflexology, into the practise and wonder of – aromaflexology!

## References:

Adamson S, Harris E, with Kerr S 1995 *The Reflexology Partnership*. The Bath Press

Adamson & Harris *The Reflexology Partnership*. Kyle C. Ltd, London

Byers D 2001 *Better Health with Foot Reflexology*. Ingham Publishing Inc, St Petersburg

Issel C 1990 *Reflexology: art, science & history*. New Frontier Publishing CA

Riley J S 1959 *Correspondence course in zone therapy reflex technique*. Mokelumne Hill CA. Page 3

Scott Byrne 2012 www. A brief history of reflexology.

O'Neil J 2016 The History of Reflexology. www.pilates4fitness.co.uk/history_of_reflexology.htm

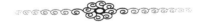

Aromaflexology

# Chapter One
# Aromaflexology

Having practised reflexology for several years alongside aromatherapy, I had, for some time, been wishing that somehow, movement was possible in a reflexology treatment. However, movement was not allowed by Doreen Bayly (who brought the Eunice Ingham method of reflexology to the UK in 1966/7) or indeed, by any other teacher of the therapy, apart from caterpillaring and circling on the spot. As a person who uses her hands when talking, I was finding the restrictions of using only pressure difficult (and – dare I say it – a bit boring).

Whilst wondering how I could introduce movement into the treatment and still have gratifying results for the patient, it was in Switzerland, in 1987, that the idea of a different technique for the treatment of foot reflexes came to me. I was giving my husband a reflexology treatment for his bronchial asthma (which had resurfaced) and decided, as well as introducing movement, to put essential oils in a base cream to see if the latter would hasten his recovery. The results after three days were more impressive than when I'd used pure reflexology previously, so I resolved to develop the technique. On returning home, I wrote notes about it and included the teaching of it on my aromatherapy courses.

I named it Swiss Reflex Treatment because of where I was when I first thought of it, under which name it was known for 27 years. However, in 2013 it came to my knowledge that both students and practitioners thought the treatment was actually a Swiss one which had been adapted for teaching in England. Because of the confusion this was causing to students, my husband Len and I (now retired) decided that the name should be changed. The name chosen was **Aromaflexology**, which, it has to be admitted, is a more professional name, especially considering it is not a Swiss treatment and that essential oils are included!

Both traditional reflexology and aromaflexology are gentle, uncomplicated treatments which encourage the body to restore itself to good health. In the former, the thumb and/

7

or fingers are applied to specific reflex points with pressure (plus a pencil in Sweden – see Introduction p. 4); in aromaflexology, the whole problematic area is massaged with a non-oily cream (to enable movement over the skin, yet having a certain amount of resistance) containing 10% of the relevant essential oils to help the client's problem/s. The percentage is high because of the very small amount of cream which is applied.

## Aromaflexology - What is it?

Although aromaflexology uses the foot reflexes, it should not be confused with reflexology; the former is carried out using essential oils and movement – the latter is not. In aromaflexology, after the first treatment by a therapist, daily treatment (by self, family member or friend) is an absolute requirement for the best results; because of this, improvement becomes evident after quite a short time. Therapists trained in aromaflexology by Shirley Price Aromatherapy, the Penny Price Academy and several other aromatherapy schools have had some extraordinarily positive results with their clients, especially on spinal problems – see Chapter Eight.

Aromaflexology is a very efficient treatment which encourages the body to return to good health in a shorter time than with reflexology. The differences between this therapy and reflexology are explained below and in the following chapters. Aromaflexology is simpler to carry out than reflexology, but it is nevertheless essential that the position of each reflex point is known by the therapist. As with all practical subjects, attending a hands-on course is the best way to learn.

Whilst this book is written for therapists, many people have a natural talent for some practical subjects, e.g. cookery. Although reflexology treatments should only be carried out by a fully trained reflexologist, it is possible, where natural talent is evident, for friends, relatives or carers who have given a therapist's clients their daily treatments, to help themselves and their loved ones with aromaflexology in the home.

However, they would only be successful if the instructions in this book were followed very carefully including – importantly – showing the person they are helping how to treat themselves daily.

Giving treatments to the general public however, requires a professional qualification in the subject.

The main differences between the treatment of foot reflexes by an aromaflexologist and that by a reflexologist are as follows:

In aromaflexology:
- the pressure is spread over a larger area rather than on one specific point at a time. This makes it possible to treat more than one reflex at the same time, when necessary.
- essential oils are added to a base resistant enough not to slip over the skin. Vegetable oil is therefore not an option – a cream base is needed with just the right amount of resistance.

In addition, I felt it was essential:
- to find a way of helping people to help themselves, thus enabling them not only to take part in their own healing, but also to enable their health to improve more rapidly than is possible with weekly visits. This is achieved by the after-care treatment being done every day.
- to make the therapy possible (as well successful) for people who couldn't afford a weekly visit to a reflexologist.

## The Object of Aromaflexology

Although based on pressure on the foot reflexes, aromaflexology differs from reflexology in several ways:
- in the assessment (Chapter Three), it uses a question and answer technique together with the foot reflexes, which are pressed individually just long enough to see if the client has a reaction, thus being able to assess the health of the client and ascertain whether or not there is a disorder present.
- having determined the possible health imbalances by this method, essential oils are added to a bland cream base – selected for each individual client, to help relieve the main (and possibly a secondary) health imbalance.
- the troubled reflexes are massaged in circular movements (see Pressure on p. 49) over specific areas, using a very small amount of the cream together with the techniques described in Chapter Four; this procedure is able to treat the body via the energy lines which flow from each reflex to the organ it represents.

Aromaflexology involves client participation – including teaching the client how to carry out a treatment on him/herself daily at home, or, if this is not possible, showing a partner or carer how to do this. It is crucial to the success of the treatment that this is done conscientiously *every day* (by self-treatment or another person). With daily participation, improvement is fairly rapid, giving faster results than would a weekly reflexology treatment, with the bonus of being less costly.

## Stress

A certain amount of stress is healthy, but when it continues for a long time without relief it can become destructive; tense muscles, which restrict the flow of necessary blood to the organs, can lead to a state of distress in which disease can develop (Adamson & Harris p.11). Unhappy emotions may also cause this imbalance, with the possibility of triggering physical dis–ease (discomfort) (Price 2000).

Rigidity in either the body or the feet usually indicates the presence of tension or stress and by easing this through massage and manipulation it can be relieved. For example, tension in the neck and shoulders indicates the presence of stress, implying the importance of massaging these areas (Stormer 2003). Thus when aromaflexology is given to someone who is stressed, it is a good idea to follow the treatment by a neck and shoulder massage with essential oils (see Chapter Seven); this has been proved to give an immediate benefit to the client (Price & Price 2012).

## Healthy Blood Circulation

The principle of good health is when all bodily systems are behaving as nature intended, complementing one another in order to balance the body. The human body, apart from its more mysterious attributes (like the ability to think – and put thoughts into words) is an intricate machine, "oiled" by the blood. As a healthy blood circulation is key to all bodily functions, it is of prime importance that the flow is unimpeded throughout the body, which it can only achieve in a *relaxed, healthy body*.

If there is congestion in the body the circulation is poor; this congestion can be caused by tension or stress – in which case health disorders can sometimes follow, as the organs do not receive enough blood and nutrients via the arteries, nor get rid of toxins via the veins. When distress occurs, the healthy circulation is interfered with, resulting eventually in unhealthy organs, represented by a blockage in the reflex points. Every organ and every part of the body needs a correct blood-flow speed in order to be completely healthy.

## How to Recognise a Blockage

When there is a malfunction (for any reason) in the blood circulation, it flows more slowly; this in turn affects the nearest organs. A blockage occurs in the energy pathway, sometimes causing crystalline deposits to form at the foot reflex point representing the organ where the disorder is showing itself. It is not really known whether these deposits are in the blood circulation at the changeover from arteries to veins, or at the nerve endings, but they can be broken down by correct pressure massage. Sometimes the blockage shows itself by the patient experiencing pain when pressure is applied. Either way, treatment using correct pressure massage brings relief from the symptoms being suffered, by unblocking the energy flow and therefore bringing about relaxation – plus relief from the symptoms being suffered.

If these crystalline deposits occur, they can sometimes be felt by a therapist as grittiness (often referred to as crystals), rather like a beanbag filling under the skin. The feeling experienced by the client varies from a strange unpleasant feeling to a sharp knife-like pain. It is important that the therapist's eyes watch the client's face carefully all the time whilst working, so that any visible reaction can be noted. If crystals are present, but the therapist cannot feel any grittiness, the expression on the client's face, plus questions, is the all-important feedback needed to enable that therapist to give an assessment of the client's health. The first time a client experiences pressure on a blocked reflex, the pain felt may be quite sharp or acute. This does not necessarily indicate a severe disorder and may be caused either by:
• stress or tension in that person.

- working beyond the client's pain threshold – never good!
   If the patient is not relaxed, but is tense, then the treatment will be ineffective.
   To summarise, blockages show their presence in three ways:
- Crystals, which when present, can be felt by the operator. Sometimes it is easier to detect the crystals when the thumb is made to slide over a small area with pressure. A good example of this is sliding along the ureter tube with pressure, from the kidney reflex to the bladder reflex.
- Client's facial reactions, which is why the therapist should watch the person's face intently all the time he/she is working on a reflex.
- Spoken feedback – achieved by the specific (and imperative) questions posed by the therapist.

## Related Areas and Reflexes

Just as organs in the body are often positioned over one another, or overlapping in some way, so are the reflexes which represent them. When there is a reaction, say, on the stomach reflex, it may be the pancreas which has the problem; similarly, part of the left lung overlaps the heart and part of the transverse colon overlaps with the kidney, etc. Thus one has to be very careful when asking questions about a reaction – and even more careful when responding to the answers, so as not to frighten the client unnecessarily. Should the therapist suspect there is something serious present, he/she should refer that person to his or her medical practitioner. In such cases it is better to talk about general areas rather than specific points, and not to state exactly what one thinks may be the problem.

## Important Points to Remember

The following important points must be remembered before carrying out either an assessment or a treatment:

1 Do not forget to note on the assessment form which reflexes have an uncomfortable reaction (confirmed by the client as being problematic) and therefore which systems will need treatment.
2 Do not confuse the assessment with a treatment – it is *not* a treatment; it is simply a means of discovering any health imbalances which may require treatment.
3 As you look at the soles of the feet in front of you, the client's right foot is on your *left* and his/her left foot is on your *right*.
4 Refer to Chapter Two if you need to be reminded of the position of any reflex.
   The wonderful thing about aromaflexology is that all tender areas can be treated without any risk of harmful effects, thus beneficial results can be obtained – *even if the exact organ requiring treatment cannot be pinpointed*. This is because an *area* is being treated rather than a specific reflex point being pressed. So... Let's find out more!

**References:**

Adamson S, Harris E 1995 *The Reflexology Partnership*. Kyle C. Ltd, London

Price 1991 *Aromatherapy for Common Ailments*. Gaia Books Ltd, London.

Price L, Price S *Aromatherapy for Health Professionals*. Churchill Livingstone, Edinburgh

Price S. 2000 *Aromatherapy for Your Emotions*. Thorsons, London

Stormer C 1995 *Reflexology- the definite guide*. Hodder& Stoughton, London

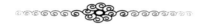

# Chapter Two
# Position of Reflex Points

O ur bodily organs are represented in the soles and upper parts of our feet in exactly the same place as they occur in our bodies. To illustrate this point clearly, take a look at the picture of the soles of the feet on page 14.

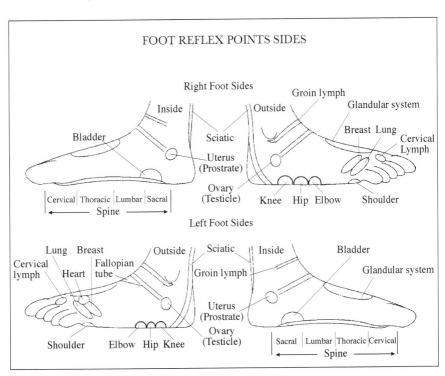

FOOT REFLEX POINTS SIDES

Right Foot Sides

Inside
Outside
Groin lymph
Glandular system
Bladder
Sciatic
Breast  Lung
Cervical Lymph
Uterus (Prostrate)
Ovary (Testicle)
Knee  Hip  Elbow
Shoulder

| Cervical | Thoracic | Lumbar | Sacral |

Spine

Left Foot Sides

Lung  Breast
Outside
Sciatic
Inside
Bladder
Cervical lymph
Fallopian tube
Heart
Groin lymph
Glandular system
Uterus (Prostrate)
Ovary (Testicle)
Shoulder  Elbow  Hip  Knee

| Sacral | Lumbar | Thoracic | Cervical |

Spine

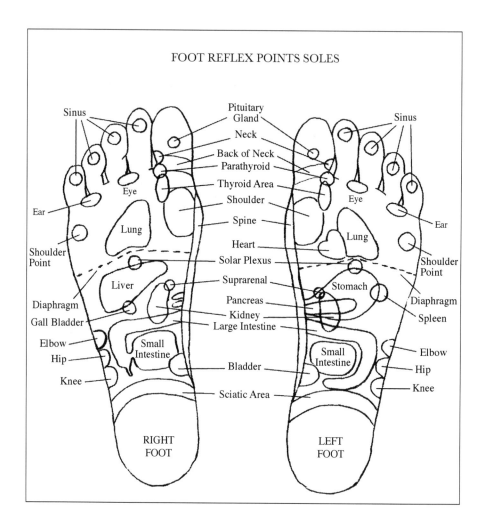

FOOT REFLEX POINTS SOLES

Looking at the two feet close together (above), it can be seen that they loosely map the anatomical layout of the whole human body.

- The two big toes put together represent the head, the neck being represented by the neck of the big toes – below the soft cushions.
- Whichever organs are on the left side of the body are only on the left foot, those on the right side of the body being only on the right foot. Thus the liver reflex is on the right foot and the heart on the left one.

- The spine is in the centre of the body; therefore, the spinal reflexes are represented down the inside edge of both feet – even the shape corresponds to the spine as seen from the side.
- The elbow reflex is halfway down the outside of the foot – a little bone can be felt there.
- As you look along the foot pad below the toes, the shoulder point is on the outside of the foot.
- The lungs are situated above the waist in the body, thus the lung reflexes are above the waistline of the feet.
- The digestive system is more complicated – see the bullet point above 'Nervous system' below.

If you look at the two feet together, it is easy to see that there is a waistline at around the middle of the feet. All the organ above the waist are represented in the area above this midline and all those organs below the waist are represented below the midline of the foot.

- When the arms are straight down, the elbow bone is on the outside of each side of the body at the waistline. The elbow reflex is very easy to find as a bony protuberance on the outside of the foot at its waist level.
- We have two kidneys, almost on the waist (or just below) and near the centre of the back. The kidney reflexes are therefore almost on the waist of the foot and situated towards its inside edge.

I could continue, but I'm sure I've made my point – if the positions of all the systems and organs in the body are known, the reflexes for them can be located without too much difficulty on the feet.

The drawings on pages 13 and 14 show where each foot reflex can be found:
- Some are on the right foot and some on the left one.
- The stomach, pancreas and kidney reflexes on the left foot overlap, so when one is treated, the whole area receives treatment.
- The spinal reflex is very long, so the cervical, thoracic and lumbar areas are treated in turn.
- To treat the digestive system as a whole, the therapist has to move from one foot to the other, as the liver and stomach are on separate feet and the small and large intestines are divided between both feet.

## 1. Nervous system

### *Solar plexus*
In the body, in the hollow just below the diaphragm, is where we often feel stress. Feel the shape of your rib cage, which rises to a peak in the middle of the chest at the sternum. The hollow just below this is the celiac or solar plexus.

To find the reflex on yourself, put one foot onto your opposite knee and your fingers round the front of your toes. You will see that the bottom of the ball of your foot is shaped exactly like a rib cage – higher in the middle. Let your thumb drop into the hollow just under the bone – this hollow is the solar plexus reflex.

### Sciatic nerve

This is a tricky one, but ask someone who suffers from sciatica and they will tell you that the pain goes from the centre of the spine across the lower back and down the leg to the little toe.

Thus, the reflex is found across the foot along the top of the heel cushion, progressing down its outside edge.

## 2. Glandular system

### Pituitary gland

This important gland is at the base of the brain – in the centre of the head, and as the reflex is situated in the centre of the lower part of big toe cushion, it is easy to locate.

### Parathyroid

This gland is situated below the pituitary gland, almost in the neck, but as it is very close to the thyroid gland, it is not easy to distinguish the reflex from that of the thyroid.

### Thyroid

In the body the area of the thyroid gland overlaps with that of the parathyroid gland. However, as the area below the parathyroid is thyroid related, it is used to represent the thyroid gland and is located in the groove just below the parathyroid reflex.

NB: The thymus, a gland concerned with the immune system, is also situated in this groove.

### Adrenal

As the adrenal gland is at the top inside edge of kidney, the reflex is easier to locate when assessing the kidney reflex (see no. 6 below).

## 3. Sinuses

In the body, these are found along the top of the cheekbones, on either side of the nose. Their reflexes are located in the centre of the cushion of each of the four small toes, as the four smaller toes are regarded as being part of the head.

### Eyes

Although in the body the eyes are above the sinuses, the reflexes are located *below* the sinus reflexes. I know of no explanation for this, but – there are exceptions to every rule!

The eye reflexes are situated in the hollow between the second and third toes, just above the ball of the foot, but just *below* the necks of the toes.

### Ears

Although the ears are level with the cheekbones, the ear reflexes, like those of the eyes, are also below the sinus reflexes. They are situated in the hollow between the fourth and fifth toes, just above the ball of the foot, but just *below* the necks of the toes.

## 4. Bone and muscular system

### Spine

The spine is all the way down the centre of the body and it can easily be seen that the curve of the foot relates to the natural curve of the spine. Because the two feet together represent the body, the spinal reflexes are on the inside edges of both feet, commencing just after the neck of the big toe and going all the way down the inside to the base of the foot.

### Neck

The neck joins the with the shoulders and because the head (as represented on the feet) is made up of the two big toes together, the neck reflex goes all the way around both toes. The inside edges are where the neck joins the shoulders.

When stressed, tension often shows itself as pain in the shoulder muscles, but can also be accompanied by discomfort in the neck when turning the head. The reflex for neck tension is on the *inside* edges of the neck of the big toes. A headache may also show itself there, or, it may show itself at the top of the cushions of the big toes, which represent the forehead.

### Shoulders

Because the shoulders are level with the base of the neck in the body, the reflexes are found along the ball of the foot just below the toes. The shoulder blade area (scapula) is found in the fleshy cushion just under the big toe, the outside edge (clavicle) being just below the neck of the little toe.

### Elbows

The arms are on the outer sides of the body, and when they are lowered, the elbows are approximately level with the waist. The elbow reflex can therefore be found by

**17**

sliding the thumb or finger down the outer side of each foot until you come to a small bony protuberance near the waist of the foot – this is the elbow reflex. (I love showing people this reflex!)

### Hips and knees
The hips and knees are on the outsides of the body, thus their reflexes are located on the outside edges of the feet. The hip reflex can be found in the little hollow just below the elbow reflex – press on this and your finger or thumb will fall into the hollow. The knee reflex is in the same hollow, but a little below the hip reflex.

## 5. Respiratory system

### Lungs
The lungs are situated behind the rib cage, protected by this and the shoulder blades. The lung reflexes are located in the ball of each foot in a fairly large area.

## 6. Excretory system

### Kidney
The kidneys are situated at around waist level on the body, on each side of the spine. Their reflexes are located around the waist level of the feet, slightly towards the inside edge. NB: The adrenal gland is above the inside edge of the kidney.

### Ureter
The ureter is the tube which carries urine from the kidney to the bladder. The reflex is easily followed by sliding down from the kidney reflex to the bladder reflex.

### Bladder
The bladder is situated centrally in the lower body. The reflex is therefore located on the inside edge of each foot, near the top of the heel. It is usually easy to find as very often there is a small round, soft raised area on the foot.

## 7. Digestive system
This is the most complicated part of the body when working on foot reflexes, as different organs are responsible for carrying out each step of the process – some

of these are on the left side of the body and some on the right side. As some of these overlap other parts of the body (for example, the stomach lies over part of the kidney), the questioning is most important when assessing the client.

Naturally, the reflexes also overlap, but using the aromaflexology technique means that you are always confident that treating the area will have the effect you were hoping for.

### Liver

The liver, a giant, almost right-angled triangular organ is situated on the right-hand side of the body, immediately below the diaphragm, the longest side going across the area just underneath it, the shorter side being parallel with, and next to, the outer side of the body. (The hypotenuse runs from bottom right to top left).

The reflex is therefore located on the right foot, found just under the ball of the foot, to the left of the solar plexus. Its rising edge is on the outer side of the foot, the longest going across the bottom of the diaphragm.

### Gall-bladder

The gall bladder is positioned near the right-hand lower edge of the liver. The reflex point overlaps the liver reflex on the right hand lower edge of the liver on the right foot.

### Pancreas

The pancreas lies behind the lower part of the stomach and is overlapped by it. The reflex lies along the lower edge of the stomach reflex and is practically covered by it. Because of this it is almost impossible to pinpoint the reflex exactly, without also touching the stomach reflex.

### Stomach

The stomach lies just below the diaphragm and starts slightly to the right of the centre of the body around waist level. Most of it is on the left side of the body.

The beginning of the stomach reflex is on the right foot, the major portion being on the left foot. It is difficult to pinpoint, as the pancreas lies in the same space. The clearest section is found underneath the ball of the left foot at the top right, level vertically in line with the fourth toe.

### Small intestine

The small intestine is situated right across the body - under both the stomach and the liver. The reflex is therefore located below the waist of each foot, from the inside edge to about three-quarters of the way towards the outside edges.

### *Ileocecal valve*

The ileocecal valve is a sphincter muscle valve which separates the small and large intestines.

It is not necessary to locate the reflex, as it is automatically passed when going from the small to the large intestines.

### *Large intestine*

The large intestine (the colon) circles practically all the way round the small intestine, from the ileocecal valve to the anus.

The ascending reflex section of the colon commences from the ileocecal valve on the outside edge of the right foot, just below the waist of the foot, above the heel cushion, going almost up to the liver reflex, just above waist level. The transverse colon reflex goes from there across to the inside edge of the right foot, continuing across the left foot to its outside edge. The descending colon reflex goes down the outside of this foot to just above the heel cushion, when it turns, to continue across the top of this, to finish at the rectum, in the centre of the foot.

## 8. Reproductive system

### *Ovaries*

The ovaries are situated at groin level, inside the body, one on each side. The reflexes are located half-way between the ankle bone and the point of heel on the outside of each foot.

### *Fallopian Tube*

This narrow tube takes eggs from the ovaries to the uterus. The reflex goes from the ovary reflex, across the top of the foot towards the inside of the ankle, where it meets the uterus reflex, half-way between the ankle bone and the point of heel on the inside of the foot.

### *Uterus*

The uterus is centrally situated in the body, between the ovaries. The reflex is located in the hollow half-way between the ankle bone and the heel edge on the inside of each foot.

## 9. Circulatory system

The blood circulation is stimulated with every reflex point which is treated, the lymph circulation being helped via the lymph reflexes. The lymphatic system has a close relationship with the blood.

### Heart

The heart is situated on the left side of the body, overlapping the lungs. It is just above the diaphragm, next to the spine and approximately level with the armpits.

It is not normally treated separately in aromaflexology, although because it overlaps the left lung it is covered when treating the lungs.

The heart reflex is located on the left foot above the "diaphragm", slightly over-lapping the spine and left lung. It can be *gently* massaged at the end of a treatment to increase the circulation in a client with poor circulation.

### Lymph

Lymph nodes are to be found in various parts of the body, the cervical nodes in the chest area and the groin being of most interest in aromaflexology.

The cervical lymph reflexes are located between toes on the *front* of the feet, as are the breast reflexes.

The groin reflexes are located just under the ankle bone on the outside of each foot.

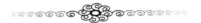

Aromaflexology

# Chapter Three
# Assessing the Client's Health

In aromaflexology, one should not try to *diagnose* the health condition of clients, although it is necessary to make an *assessment* of any problems affecting them before a treatment. An assessment is done by applying pressure to all the reflex points system by system and by *using questions* to determine any imbalances affecting their health. This questioning, which ensures client participation, is a most important part of the treatment and must be carried out with *full eye contact* between therapist and client so that any reaction to pressure can be seen clearly on the client's face.

## Preparation

1) The therapist will need to make copies of the Record Sheet (pages 46/47), by whatever means at his or her disposal.

2) The client should visit the toilet just before a treatment, to help eliminate any toxins which may be present in the urine; it also makes sure unnecessary discomfort is not felt during the assessment, perhaps leading to a false conclusion.

3) Make certain that clients being treated are sitting comfortably as it is essential for them to be as relaxed as possible. Aromaflexology can be carried out on a massage couch with:

- the head rest up so that clients can lean back comfortably on a pillow and see the therapist's face clearly.
- the therapist sitting on a chair so that he or she can also see the client's face clearly.
- a pillow under the client's knees to add to their comfort.

Alternatively, the treatment can be carried out using two chairs - the client sitting on one, and the therapist on the other, at a suitable height to reach the client's reflexes easily. The therapist should put a pillow on his or her knees on which the client's feet can rest.

If the client is not familiar with reflexology, place his or her feet together and hold the big toes together with one hand. Show, and explain to the client, how the organs of the body are mirrored in the feet, i.e. that:

- the big toes, when placed together, represent the head.
- the bony area on the inner side of each foot represents the spine.
- just as when the arms are by the side of the body, the elbow is half way down the outside of the body, the elbow reflex is halfway down the outside of the foot – a little bone can be felt there (show client).

Explain other organs in the related places in the foot – i.e. one liver (here), two kidneys (here), etc.

Complete concentration is necessary for good results; the assessment technique – and the treatment – must never be automatic. As in all contact treatments, there must be total empathy between therapist and client; when this exists, the healing energy flows from one to the other, making the benefits to the client more satisfying and lasting.

Finally, the client should breathe in a relaxed and normal manner, establishing a comfortable rhythm before treatment begins.

## Assessment – with Client Participation

Verbal participation by the person being treated is an integral and essential part of both the assessment and the treatment. This cannot be stressed enough!

During the assessment, a person's pain threshold should be discovered – and pressures on the reflexes adjusted accordingly. If clients are stressed, all points may be very sensitive, so be gentle at first, until you assess their pain threshold.

Even if they have told you their particular problem (or problems), still carry out a full assessment; another reason for their health problem may be discovered.

Assessment Questions:

As you locate and gently press a reflex, watch the person's face very carefully for a reaction. If there is no reaction, a *negative* question should be asked:

'So you don't suffer from stress?' …. (when pressing the solar plexus reflex).

'So you don't have backache very often?' …. (when pressing the spinal reflexes).

'So you have no respiratory problems?' …. (when pressing the lung reflex).

However, some people have a stronger pain threshold than others (or you may not have been quite in the right place), so they may say 'No' when there actually is a problem. This is why the questioning is so important – if there is no reaction, the answer gives the essential key to the client's health in that area.

Whenever the answer is 'Yes, I do', make a note of the nature of the problem on the record sheet.

Negatively phrased questions like the above are less worrying to the client than asking all the time 'Do you have a problem with… ?' , or 'so you suffer with …?'.

If, however, grittiness can be felt by the operator, or the client's face screws up, the questioning should be ***positive***:

'Ah! So you suffer with backache' or;

'H'mm! Your reaction suggests (or my fingers can feel) that you may have a problem connected with your lungs'. The word "***may***" is important, so as not to cause the client to become over-anxious.

When there is a reaction, the person can usually tell you what the problem is. However, if they are not aware of one, tell them only that it is possible they may have a slight imbalance in that area – which is precisely what it could be!

## Order and Method of Work for Assessment Purposes:

The following text goes through the order and method of work for the assessment technique and should be carried out, together with the questioning, as described above. For small area reflex points like the solar plexus, the tip of the bent thumb is pressed into the foot, gently at first, in case the person's pain threshold is very low. Pressure can be gradually increased until the pain threshold is reached, as if there is a problem in that part of the body, pain would be felt on the reflex itself.

On large or long reflexes (lungs and spine respectively), a technique called caterpillaring is used. Caterpillaring is when the tip of the bent thumb is placed with pressure on the beginning of the reflex. Keeping firm hold of the foot, and without moving the rest of the hand, the first joint of the thumb is lifted (which straightens it), and by flattening the joint, it moves a fraction further forward. It is bent again, the tip pressing into the next part of the reflex, then straightened once more, this sequence being repeated until the whole reflex area has been covered.

Check the reflexes representing each bodily system on *both* feet before progressing to the next system.

Always start with the foot on your left-hand side. Remember the *right* foot will be on your *left* and the *left* foot will be on your *right*!

Make notes on the record sheet whenever a health problem is confirmed by the client's reaction to your pressure – and the all-important questions.

## Introductory massage

First wipe the feet with cotton wool and an antiseptic and begin with a gentle, relaxing foot massage. Feet should always be held firmly, as it is irritating and counters relaxation to have a light 'tickly' touch on one's feet. This cannot be stressed enough, as a light touch can be very off-putting, however much someone wants to try the treatment.

1) Wrap the left foot (on your right) in a towel to keep warm, then proceed as follows on the right foot.
2) With hands facing opposite ways but close together, place them behind one another with the palms on the top of the foot (3.1M). Move both hands up to the ankle, then open them so that they are on either side of the foot (3.2M). Now moving one hand underneath the foot and the other on top, return to the toes, sandwiching the foot in between your hands (3.3M). Repeat the sequence two or three times.
3) Holding the foot firmly, rotate the ankle slowly, clockwise then anticlockwise, twice each way (3.4M).
4) Rotate the big toe gently and slowly, twice each way (3.5M).
5) Repeat step 2.
6) Wrap this foot in a towel to keep warm and repeat 2 to 5 on the right foot (the assessment begins on this foot).

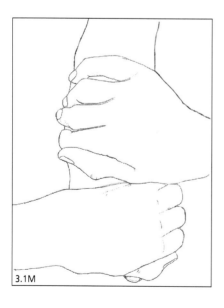

3.1M

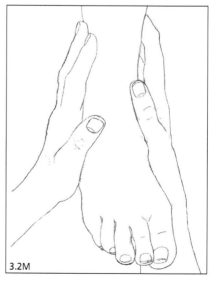

3.2M

Important points to remember:
- Do not confuse assessment with treatment – it is *not* a treatment; it is simply a means of discovering any health imbalances which may require treatment.
- As you look at the soles of the feet in front of you, the right foot is on your **left** and the left foot is on your **right**.
- If you need to be reminded of the position of any reflex, refer to Chapter Two.
- Note on the assessment form which reflexes have an uncomfortable reaction (confirmed by the client through correct questioning as being problematic).

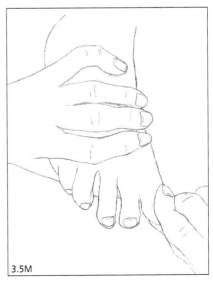

3.3M

To check the position of reflex positions on each foot, refer to the diagrams in Chapter Two, pages 13 and 14.

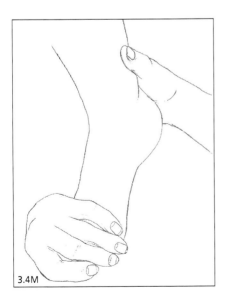

3.4M

3.5M

## 1. Nervous System

**Solar plexus** – diagram 3.1: *As the bottom of the ball of the foot represents the body's rib-cage, the solar plexus reflex can be located in the hollow just below this, in the centre.*

Hold the right foot with the left hand – fingers on the top of the foot, thumb in front, and push the toes well back. Placing the fingers of your right hand behind the foot, bend the right thumb joint and press with the side of your thumb tip into the deepest hollow under the 'rib-cage'; this is the solar plexus.

Reverse holds to locate and check this reflex on the left foot.

**Sciatic nerve** – diagram 3.2: *The sciatic nerve is located along the top of the heel cushion and down the outer edge of the heel.*

Holding the right foot with your left hand, caterpillar across the top of the heel cushion from the inside edge towards the outside of the foot with your right thumb, continuing down the outer edge of the heel to its base.

Reverse hands to locate and check this reflex on the left foot.

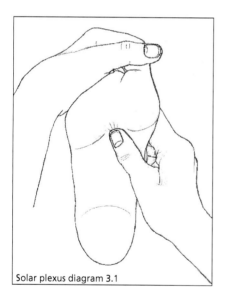

Solar plexus diagram 3.1

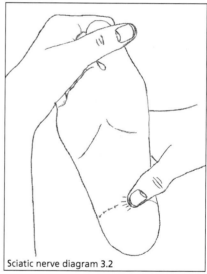

Sciatic nerve diagram 3.2

## 2. Glandular system

**Pituitary gland** – diagram 3.3: *The pituitary gland reflex point is located approximately in the centre of the big toe cushion.*

Hold the four small toes on the right foot back with the left hand. Place the fingers of the right hand behind the big toe and apply pressure on the pituitary gland reflex with the tip of your bent right thumb.

**Parathyroid** – diagram 3.4: *The parathyroid reflex is located just below the base of the big toe – almost between that and the second toe.*

Holding all the toes back with the left hand, press downwards on the reflex with the tip of your bent right thumb.

**Thyroidal area** – diagram 3.5: *As the thyroid reflex is very close to the parathyroid reflex it is difficult to be certain which of the two is being reached. For this reason, the thyroidal area,*

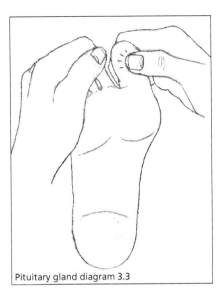

Pituitary gland diagram 3.3

*located in the groove below the space between the big and second toes, is used instead.*

Maintaining the hold above, and with the right-hand fingers behind the foot, caterpillar up the groove between and below the big and first toes with the outside of your left thumb.

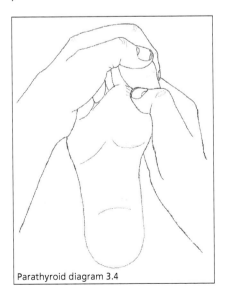

Parathyroid diagram 3.4

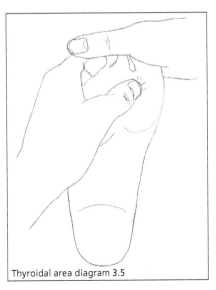

Thyroidal area diagram 3.5

29

**Adrenal gland**. See complete foot diagram.

*The adrenal reflex is located at the top inside edge of the kidney reflex, but is easier to locate when assessing the kidney (see the Excretory System below).*

Reverse hands to locate and check the glandular reflexes on the left foot.

## 3. Sinuses, Eyes and Ears

**Sinuses** – diagram 3.6: *The sinus reflexes are located in the centre of the toe cushions of the four small toes.*

Hold the side of the right foot with your right hand, fingers behind the foot, thumb in front. Placing the left hand fingers behind the toes, use the left thumb to locate each sinus point in turn – on the second to fifth toes.

NB: diagram shows the third toe.

**Eye** – diagram 3.7: *The eye reflex is located in the web between the second and third toes.*

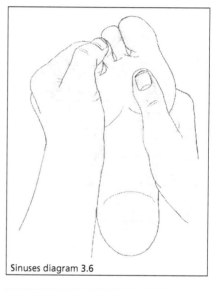

Sinuses diagram 3.6

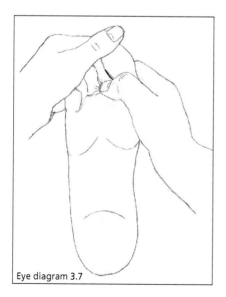

Eye diagram 3.7

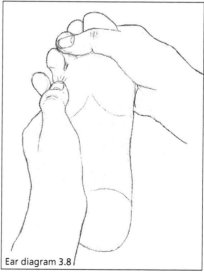

Ear diagram 3.8

Holding the right toes back with your left hand, push them back with the thumb. Place your right-hand fingers behind the foot, resting on those of the left hand and press downwards into the junction between the second and third toes with your bent right thumb tip.

**Ear** – diagram 3.8: *This reflex point is located in the web between the fourth and fifth toes.*

Now hold the right toes back with your right hand and with the fingers of the left hand behind the foot, press into the junction between the fourth and fifth toes with the tip of your bent *left* thumb.

Reverse hands to locate and check the above reflexes on the left foot.

## 4. Bone and muscular system

The curve of the inside edge of the foot relates to the natural curve of the spine in the body.

**Upper spine** – diagrams 3.9 and 3.10 (cervical and thoracic regions): *The reflex areas of the cervical and thoracic spine are found on the inner edge of the foot, from the neck of the big toe joint down to the waistline of the foot.*

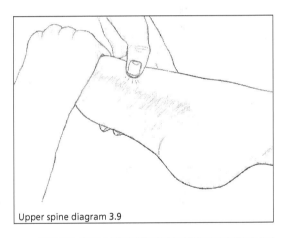

Upper spine diagram 3.9

Place your right hand over the client's toes, taking the foot over to your left (3.9). With your left fingers on the top of the foot find the channel which runs down the length of the foot's "spine" between the bone and the muscle.

Caterpillar with your left thumb down this channel as far as the waist of the foot (3.10), but not as far as bladder reflex.

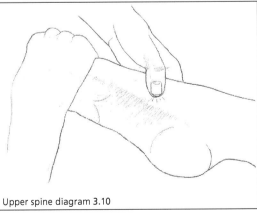

Upper spine diagram 3.10

**Lower spine** – diagram 3.11 – lumbar area: *The lumbar area reflex is located below the bladder reflex, along the edge of the heel.*

Lift the foot up slightly with your left hand around the top of the foot and place the fingers of your right hand under the heel.

Caterpillar with your right thumb from just below the bladder reflex down the edge of the heel to the base.

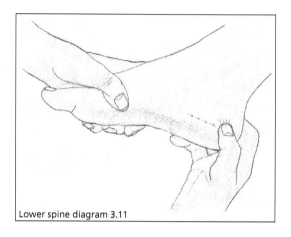

Lower spine diagram 3.11

**Neck** – diagrams 3.12, 3.13 and 3.14: *The neck reflexes are all around the neck of the big toe, the most reactive usually being on the outside of the big toe and the inner side nearest to the second toe.*

With the foot upright, hold the little toes with the left hand, grasping the big toe with the fingers of the right hand. Caterpillar all around the neck of the big toe with your right thumb (3.12 & 3.13). Change hands to check the outside edge of the neck (3.14).

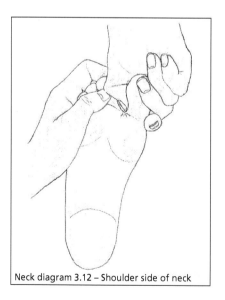

Neck diagram 3.12 – Shoulder side of neck

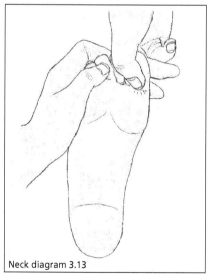

Neck diagram 3.13

**Shoulder** – diagram 3.15 (shoulder blade); 3.16 (shoulder point): *The shoulder blade reflex area is located in the fleshy part (cushion) beneath the big toe.*

Hold the top of the foot upright with your left hand (fingers behind toes), pushing the big toe back with your left thumb (3.15). Caterpillar two or three rows up the soft area below the neck of the big toe with your right thumb. This can be done in three rows (from left to right) from the base of the cushion to the neck of the toe.

*The shoulder point (outer shoulder) is located just below the neck of the little toe.*

Hold the toes with the right hand (3.16) and with the fingers of the left hand resting behind the foot, caterpillar around the bone just below the little toe with the left thumb.

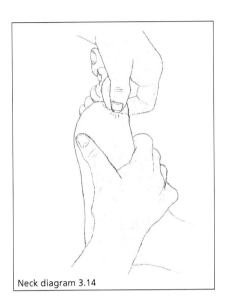

Neck diagram 3.14

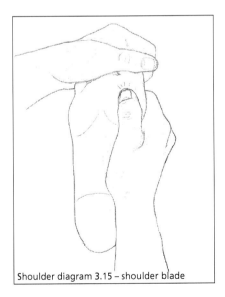

Shoulder diagram 3.15 – shoulder blade

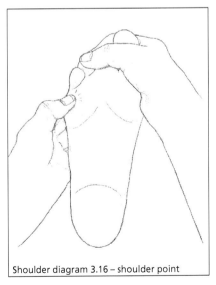

Shoulder diagram 3.16 – shoulder point

**Elbow** – diagram 3.17: *The elbow reflex is roughly halfway down the outside of the foot and is a small bony protuberance, which can be easily located.*

Holding the foot with your left hand (fingers on top of it), take it over to the right. With your right hand fingers over the top of the foot, slide your right thumb down the outside edge of the foot almost to 'waist' level (approximately halfway down) until a small bony point is found (elbow reflex). Caterpillar all around this with your thumb.

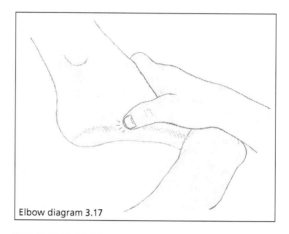

Elbow diagram 3.17

**Hip** – diagram 3.18: *The hip reflex is at the top of the hollow located immediately below the elbow reflex.*

With the hand-hold as for the elbow reflex, place your left thumb on the 'elbow bone' and slide into the top of the hollow just below it (this upper

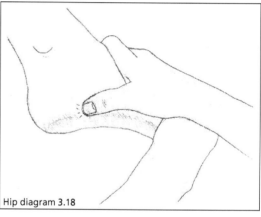

Hip diagram 3.18

part of the hollow is the hip reflex). Press inwards and upwards towards the 'elbow bone'.

**Knee** (no diagram): *The knee reflex is located in the same hollow, immediately below the hip reflex.*

Keeping the same hold, move your thumb very slightly down from the hip reflex, this time pressing inwards and downwards towards the heel bone.

Reverse hands to locate and check the spinal reflexes on the left foot.

## 5. Respiratory system

**Lungs** – diagrams 3.19 and 3.20: *The lung reflex is located on the ball of the foot.*

Hold the top of the right foot with the fingers of your left hand behind the toes as

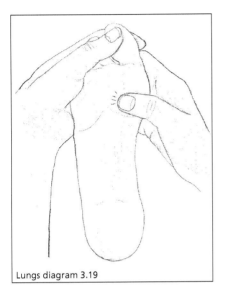

Lungs diagram 3.19

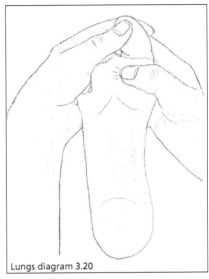

Lungs diagram 3.20

in diagram. With the fingers of your left hand resting over those of your right, caterpillar with your right thumb from the base of the ball of the foot (3.19), up towards the second toe (3.20). Moving slightly to the left, start at the base again and caterpillar up to the middle toe. Caterpillar a third row slightly to the left again, up to the fourth toe.

Reverse hands to locate and check the lung reflex on the left foot.

**6. Digestive system** (Liver, gall bladder, stomach, pancreas, small intestine, large intestine)
This is a difficult sequence to carry out, as to follow the system in the order of the digestive process it is necessary to work from the right foot, moving then to the left one, back once more to the right and finally, finishing on the left foot.

To compound matters, the pancreas and kidney reflexes overlap the stomach reflex; it is therefore difficult to know which reflex may be needing treatment. For example, there could be a reaction here if the client's kidneys are healthy but he/ she is diabetic. Thus, it can be seen that the questioning technique is very important, and should it uncover a problem, whether digestive or excretory, this can be helped successfully with aromaflexology.

**Locations of the digestive system reflexes:**
The liver is large and triangular in shape, the longest side of its reflex being on the outside of the foot.

The gall bladder reflex is also on the right foot.

Although the entrance to the stomach reflex and the start of the pancreas reflex are on the right foot, both are mainly on the left foot. On the right foot, the pancreas and kidney reflexes overlap with the bottom part of the stomach reflex (see complete foot diagram), so the act of questioning cannot be stressed enough, especially as the pancreas is not easily assessed separately from the stomach.

The spleen reflex is near the top right of the stomach reflex – see complete foot diagram.

As the small and large intestine reflexes are found on both feet, the assessment has to continue from foot to foot (also when carrying out the treatment).

**Liver** – diagrams 3.21 and 3.22: *This large reflex is located on the left-hand side of the right foot, just below the ribcage.*

Holding the toes of the right foot with your right hand as shown in diagram 3.21, caterpillar up the foot towards the fourth toe with the thumb of your left hand, starting about 1 cm in from the outside edge of the foot just above the 'waist', going up as far as the 'rib-cage'. Caterpillar up a second row, one thumb's width to the right, in line with third toe (3.22).

A further shorter row of caterpillaring can be done on the liver reflex slightly to the right of the second.

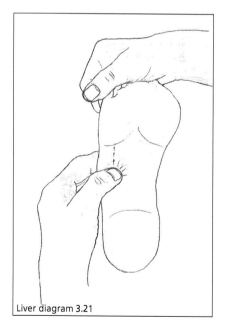
Liver diagram 3.21

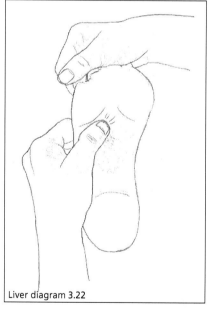
Liver diagram 3.22

**Gall bladder** – diagram 3.23: *The gall bladder is a very small reflex located at the base of the liver reflex, 2 to 3 cm from the outside edge, approximately at the centre of the foot.*

Return to the base of the liver reflex and move your thumb diagonally slightly down towards the outside edge of the foot; this is approximately where the gall bladder reflex is situated.

**Stomach** – diagram 3.24: *Stomach and pancreas – these two reflexes are located mainly on the left foot (the pancreas overlaps the bottom of the stomach reflex).*

Change over to the *left* foot, where most of this reflex is located. As explained above, the pancreas (and the kidney) overlaps with the stomach, therefore, the questioning part of the aromaflexology technique is particularly important here, i.e. "Are you diabetic?" Questions regarding the excretory system can be left till assessing the kidney-bladder reflexes.

Continuing to hold the left toes with your right hand (thumb in front), push the toes back. Caterpillar with your left thumb just above the base of the stomach reflex (left to right) and slightly above the waist level of the foot. Caterpillar a second row just above this, finishing with a slightly shorter third row (depending on the size of your client's feet). These last two rows may give a clearer reaction if there is a stomach problem, as there is less likelihood of overlapping the kidney or pancreatic reflexes.

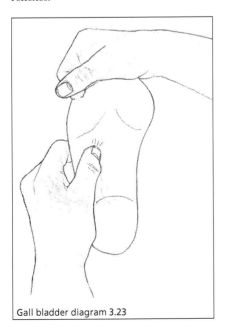

Gall bladder diagram 3.23

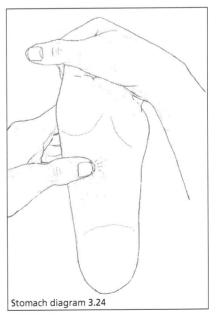

Stomach diagram 3.24

**Small intestine** – diagrams 3.25 and 3.26: *The entrance to the small intestine is on the left side of the body and therefore its reflex area is located on the left foot just below the stomach reflex, but above the base of the large intestine reflex (see complete foot diagram in Chapter Two, on pages 13 and 14).*

*As the small intestine is spread over the whole width of the body, it is necessary to complete its treatment by changing to the right foot.*

Keeping the hold above and still working on the left foot, caterpillar three horizontal rows with your left thumb in the small, soft area between the transverse colon and the base of the colon, commencing at the inside edge of the foot (3.25 shows the end of this row).

Caterpillar another row immediately below this, as close to the first one as possible, and a third immediately below the second.

Change to the *right* foot (on your left), and, holding the toes with your left hand (fingers on top of foot), caterpillar three horizontal rows with your right thumb on that half of the small intestine reflex (3.26).

**Ileocecal valve** – *this separates the small and large intestine (see complete foot diagram) and is automatically covered when continuing to the large intestine.*

The ileocaecal valve is not treated – it is just passed through on the way to the large intestine However, it is necessary to change hands to treat the large intestine.

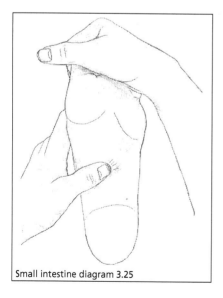

Small intestine diagram 3.25

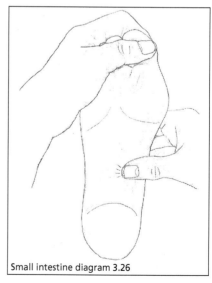

Small intestine diagram 3.26

**Large intestine** – diagrams 3.27; 3.28; 3.29 and 3.30 : *The large intestine reflex encircles the small intestine reflex.*

Still working on the right foot, hold it now with your *right* hand. Caterpillar with your left thumb through the ileocecal valve up the ascending colon reflex to the waist of the foot, then along the transverse colon to the inside edge of the foot (3.27).

As you go past the kidney there may be a reaction from that reflex.

Return to the *left* foot, holding it with your *right* hand and continue caterpillaring along the transverse colon with your *left* thumb, to the outside of that foot (3.28).

To caterpillar down the descending colon and across the last section of the large intestine, change the hand-hold, and, holding the same foot with your *left* hand, use your *right* thumb to caterpillar down the reflex, then across to the inside edge of the foot (3.29).

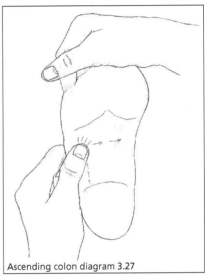

Ascending colon diagram 3.27

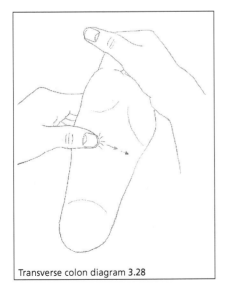

Transverse colon diagram 3.28

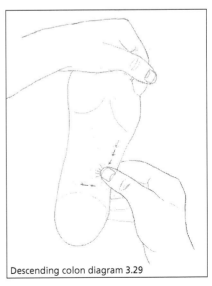

Descending colon diagram 3.29

**39**

To complete the large intestine as far as the anus, continue to caterpillar across the foot with your right thumb, up to the inside edge of the foot, which finishes the complex digestive system (3.30).

## 7. Excretory system

(Kidney, ureter tube and bladder)
The kidney reflex is located just above the waist level of the foot, about one third in from the inside edge and diagonally down from solar plexus, towards the inside edge of the foot.

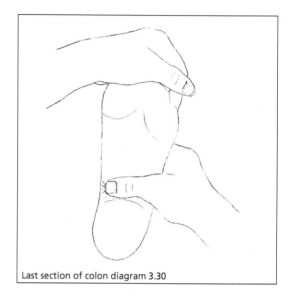

Last section of colon diagram 3.30

The bladder reflex is very often a little raised area on the inside edge of the foot below the 'waist', just below the bottom of the thoracic spinal reflex.

The ureter tube reflex goes diagonally from the kidney to the bladder.

**Kidney and bladder** – diagrams 3.31 and 3.32: *It is easier to find the kidney reflex if the bladder reflex is found first. So ……*

Place your right hand over the client's toes and take the foot over to your left. With your left-hand fingers on top of the foot (i.e. behind it), find the bladder reflex (see above), lightly place your left thumb on it – without pressure, and slide it gently diagonally upwards and slightly inwards along the ureter tube reflex until the kidney reflex is reached (3.31).

Most people have a reaction when this reflex is pressed, as this is where toxins gather before being

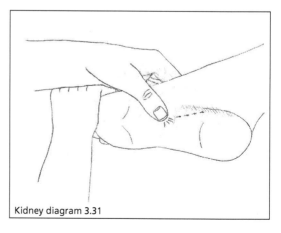

Kidney diagram 3.31

eliminated; this is one reason why it is good to ask the client to go to the toilet before commencing the treatment.

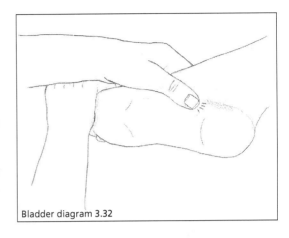

Bladder diagram 3.32

Should there be a reaction, the above should be explained to the client, and be followed by the question "I assume you don't have any problems with your kidneys". If there *does* happen to be a problem, the client will then tell you about it.

After putting pressure on the kidney reflex with your thumb, caterpillar down the ureter tube, finishing on the bladder reflex (3.32).

(NB. The adrenal gland is on the top inside edge of the kidney.)

Reverse hands to locate and check the reflexes on the left foot.

## 8. Reproductive system

**Ovaries** – diagram 3.33:

*The ovary reflex is located on the outside of the foot exactly halfway between the point of the heel and the ankle bone on the outside edge of the foot.*

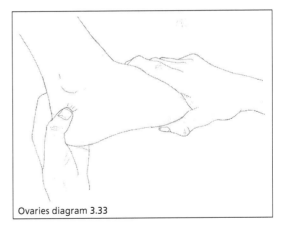

Ovaries diagram 3.33

Place the fingers of your right hand over the toes (thumb over little toe) and take the foot over to the right.

Cradle the heel with your left palm and press lightly on the ovary reflex with your left thumb.

**41**

**Fallopian Tube** – diagrams 3.34 and 3.35: *The fallopian tube reflex is located across the top of the foot, going from the ovaries to the uterus.*

Keeping the same hold, caterpillar with your left thumb from the ovary across the top of the foot, to the other ankle bone, turning the foot gently towards you as you reach the middle.

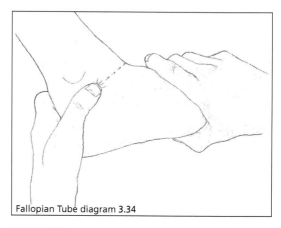

Fallopian Tube diagram 3.34

**Uterus** – diagram 3.36
*The uterus reflex is located on the inside of the foot, exactly halfway between the point of the heel and the ankle bone on the inside of the foot.*

Place your right hand over the toes (thumb on ball of foot) and take it over to the left. Placing the fingers of your left hand across the top of the foot press the uterus reflex. As this reflex is often sensitive, begin with a gentle pressure.

Reverse hands to locate and check the reflexes on the left foot.

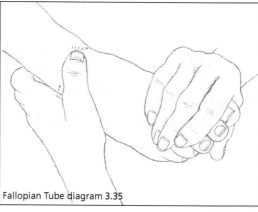

Fallopian Tube diagram 3.35

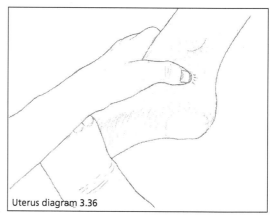

Uterus diagram 3.36

## 9. Circulatory system

Every reflex point pressed helps to increase circulation to a certain extent and can also help to prevent blockage in the arteries, veins and valves.

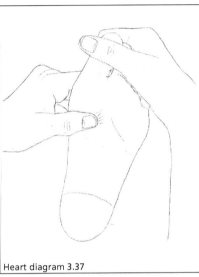

Heart diagram 3.37

**Heart** – diagram 3.37: *The heart reflex, which is on the left foot only, slightly to the left of the solar plexus, is rarely touched during an aromaflexology treatment, but can be **lightly** massaged at the end of a treatment if the person has a suspected heart problem.*

NB: If you are present when someone suffers a heart attack, the heart reflex may be massaged gently whilst waiting for the ambulance to arrive.

Place your right hand over the toes of the left foot, fingers on top of the foot (3.37) to locate the heart reflex with the left thumb.

**Cervical lymph** – diagrams 3.38 and 3.39: *The cervical lymph reflexes are located on the front of the foot in the hollows between and below the toes.*

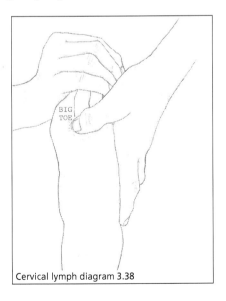

Cervical lymph diagram 3.38

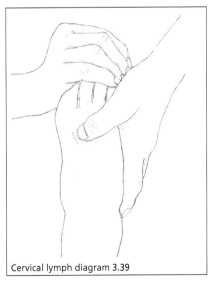

Cervical lymph diagram 3.39

**43**

With the right hand fingers over the front of the toes of the right foot, bend the latter towards you. Placing the fingers of the left hand along the side of the foot, use the thumb to caterpillar down the spaces between the first and second toes, second and third toes and third and fourth toes.

**Groin lymph** – diagram 3.40
*The groin lymph is located around the back of the ankle bone*

Place the fingers of your right hand over the toes, taking the foot over to the right. Cradling the heel with your left palm, caterpillar around the ankle bone with your thumb.

Reverse hand-holds to locate and check the lymphatic reflexes on the left foot.

NB: The lymphatic system is included here because of its close relationship to the blood circulation.

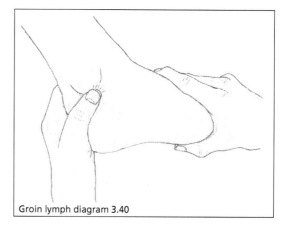

Groin lymph diagram 3.40

After completing the client assessment (making all necessary notes on the client record card), select the essential oils which will give the most benefit to the client. Details of how to do this are at the beginning of Chapter Four.

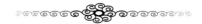

# Chapter Four

# Treatment of Painful Reflexes

As explained in Chapter One, in order to show improvement in health problems presented it is important that the treatment be carried out every day and the regular, everyday stimulation of the reflexes ensures this. If clients are unable to carry out self-treatment (see Chapter Six, page 61), they should bring to the appointment their partner, carer or friend (someone able to give daily treatments), to be shown exactly how to carry these out.

## Preparation for Home Treatment

The partner, carer or friend should be given a seat where the therapist's hands at work can easily be seen, as after the treatment, they will be carrying out the same routine, under the supervision of the therapist. At the following appointment, they will be asked to go through the treatment, to make sure their movements and sequence are correct.

## Treatment Technique

During an assessment technique the client's problem areas are detected by pressing firmly on the relevant reflexes (or caterpillaring on a large one). However, during a treatment, *the whole reflex area is massaged* with the thumb, in circular movements, with pressure on the first half of the circle and relaxing on the return half.

## Selecting the Essential Oils

The method by which the essential oils are selected for each client is important in order to obtain the best results.

Having ascertained the state of the client's health through the assessment, write, at the top of column one on the record sheet, the client's main health anxiety. At the top of the second column, enter the next most important consideration and should there be something else the client would like help with, even if not top priority, write this at the top of the third column.

# AROMAFLEXOLOGY RECORD SHEET

| Therapists name: | Case number: | |
|---|---|---|
| Client Name: | Occupation: | |
| Address: | Tel (home): | Tel (work): |
| | D.O.B.: | Children?: |
| | Height/weight: | |

| Diet/Allergies/Sensitivities?: |
|---|
| Smoking/Alcohol?: |
| Medical History: |
| Medication: |
| Side Effects: |

| Exercise: | Interests: |
|---|---|
| Family History: | |
| Signature: | Date: |

| First Condition | | | Second condition | | | Third condition | | |
|---|---|---|---|---|---|---|---|---|
| | | | | | | | | |
| | | | | | | | | |
| | | | | | | | | |
| | | | | | | | | |
| | | | | | | | | |
| | | | | | | | | |
| | | | | | | | | |
| | | | | | | | | |
| | | | | | | | | |

Essential oils chosen (drops):

Home treatment plan:

## REFLEX INDICATIONS

Nervous:

Glandular:

Respiratory:

Muscle/Skeletal:

Renal:

Digestive:

Reproductive:

Lymphatic:

Precautions:

Comments and advice:

## And Now – The Choice!

1) Look up in Chapter Nine the essential oils which could help the client's main condition and list five or six of these in the first column of the record sheet.
2) In the second column, list the essential oils which could help the client's second most important problem.
3) Should there be a third condition troubling the client, write down the oils which could help this in the third column.

If essential oils in the first column are repeated in the second one, underline these *in column one*. Should an essential oil in column three be in column one, underline this – also in column one – but with a *dotted* line this time, to show that it is to aid a less severe problem.

If any oils in the third column are in column two, underline them *in column two*.

The total number of drops normally added to 30 ml of base cream is 30 (see Notes below).

The oils selected for use should all come from the first column, where there are oils underlined from the other two columns. To the cream, add the highest number of drops from those oils which are underlined from column two; the lowest from those underlined from column three. Thus the proportions of the blend will be in proportion to the needs of the client.

If there are no repeats from columns two or three, the highest number of drops should be taken from three of the essential oils in column one, with a lesser number taken from an oil in column two. If there is a third condition, an even lower number of drops can be added from this column if felt to be needed.

*Notes:*
- *Poor circulation is helped automatically throughout an aromaflexology treatment, but check to see if any of the oils to aid this already occur in one of the columns.*
- *If the client is suffering from high blood pressure, up to 10 drops of the relevant essential oils can be added to the 30 being used to help the client's main health problem/s - i.e. up to 40 drops can be used in total. As such a very tiny amount of cream is needed for a treatment, there is no risk of essential oil overuse.*

## Treatment

During a first treatment, any pain felt may be quite sharp or acute – this does not necessarily indicate a severe disorder and may be caused by:
- Tension in the client – if the patient is not relaxed, the treatment will not be so effective.
- The therapist working beyond the client's pain threshold – never good!
- Incorrect pressure. Pressure should be relevant to the client's pain threshold, and having found this, it should be maintained throughout the treatment of that particular reflex area. A couple of minutes on each troubled reflex area is usually enough at any one treatment.

### *Important points to remember*

Treatment should *always* begin with the solar plexus reflex, whether or not it was discovered during the assessment that the client was stressed or anxious. This should be followed by all reflexes which were shown in the assessment to be requiring treatment (whether by reaction or questioning). The treatment should *always* finish with the kidney-ureter-bladder reflexes, whether or not a problem was indicated in the assessment, to help take toxins to the bladder, ready for excretion.

- Complete concentration must be given to the job in hand, with no extraneous thoughts in the mind of the therapist.
- The assessment technique in Chapter Three and the treatment which follows must never be automatic, i.e. without showing consideration for the client.
- A couple of minutes on each troubled reflex is usually enough to give in one treatment. No reflex should be treated for longer than this; if the pain has not abated in that time, check that, when commencing on that reflex, you were not applying pressure above the client's pain threshold. Remember, watching the client's face for reaction and taking heed of a severe wince, is the best way of determining if you are overdoing the pressure. However, don't forget that *some* discomfort should be felt on a problematic reflex.
- As previously stated (Chapter Three), the feet should always be held in a firm grip, as a light touch is a bit like a loose handshake and is not only uncomfortable but also prevents people from completely relaxing.
- The location and hand-holds for treatment are exactly the same as for the assessment.
- The reflexes for each troubled system should be located and treated on *both* feet (as in the assessment), before moving to the next system.
- If the client found it painful in the stomach area in the assessment, or questioning uncovered a problem, reflexes for the *whole* of the digestive system should be treated.

### *Thumbs*

Thumbs are the main 'tools' used in carrying out an aromaflexology treatment, most movements being done with the side of the thumb (outside edge) in the form of a circle.

It is essential that the thumb nails are very short, especially on the outer edge.

### *Pressure*

The pressure applied to a reflex on the first half of the massage circling is of the utmost importance, too little being insufficient to give a reaction on the reflex, too much being suddenly too painful on a tender one (sensitive people react more quickly). However, the pressure should always be sufficient to cause the client some discomfort, in order to note any change.

The return half of the circle should always be light.

Using the correct amount of pressure during circling determines the amount of healing taking place in the client.

### Treating a large area

For a large area like the spine, lungs, etc. treat small areas at a time, until the whole reflex has been covered.

### Empathy

As in all contact treatments, including aromatherapy, there must be total empathy between operator and recipient; when this exists, the healing energy flows from one to the other, making the benefits more satisfying and lasting.

### Hand positions (Hand-holds)

Remember that hand positions for the right foot should be reversed for treating the left foot.

### Eye contact

While massaging all reflex areas and questioning the client, it is very important to look at the client's face the whole time – not at what you are doing.

The questions to be asked during the progression of the massage are below and should be carried out diligently in order to obtain the best results.

### Client Comfort

- Check that the client is still comfortable and is not in need of the toilet.
- If the client is not relaxed, the first treatment can commence with the following preliminary foot massage movements to induce a relaxed condition.

### Pre-Treatment Massage

1) Starting with the left foot (on your *right!*), apply a small amount of cream over the whole of the foot.
2) With hands facing opposite ways but close together, place them behind one another with the palms on the top of the foot (4aM).

Take the hands firmly up to the ankle, then open them so that they are on either side of the foot (4bM).

Moving one hand underneath the foot and the other on top, return to the toes, sandwiching the foot in between your hands with pressure (4cM)

3) Repeat this two or three times, then wrap the foot in a towel
4) Repeat on the right foot.

Begin the treatment on this foot. (4dM) (4eM, 4fM – see pp. 51-52).

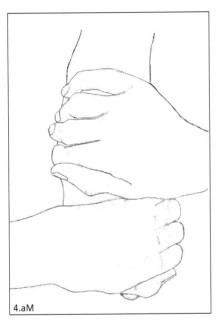

4.aM

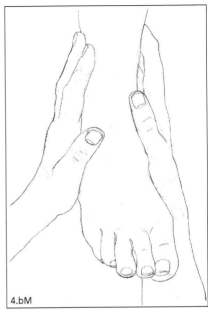

4.bM

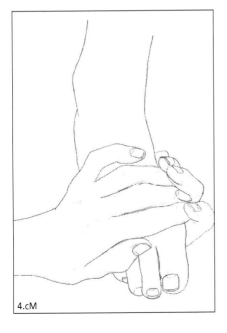

4.cM

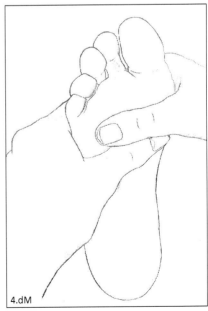

4.dM

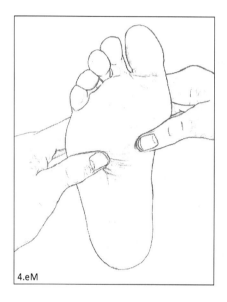
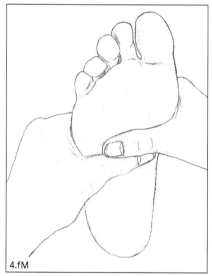

4.eM

4.fM

### *Treatment of troubled reflexes*

Treatment should:

- start with the solar plexus reflex area to encourage relaxation.
- finish with the excretory system reflex areas to encourage elimination of toxins.

In between these, treat the troubled reflexes, always starting with the right foot (on your left) before treating the left foot (on your right), completing treatment on that system before passing to the next one requiring treatment.

Troubled systems should be treated in the same order as they occur in the assessment, e.g. glandular; sinuses, eyes and ears; spinal column, lungs, etc. and each one treated on both feet before beginning on the next system. This keeps up the continuity of related reflexes and also helps maintain equilibrium and relaxation in the body.

### *Treatment questions*

The following questions are equally as important as the assessment questions.

***Keep your eyes on the client all the time***, whilst asking the following:

'Is the pain reducing at all?' Repeat the question after a few seconds.

After several seconds of working on the area, the person may say (incredulously!): 'Yes – it's not as painful; are you pressing as hard as you were before?'

Having assured them that the pressure has always been the same, you now say: 'I want you to tell me when the pain has nearly gone.'

Then you ask: 'Has it gone yet?' When the pain has completely gone, treatment on that reflex is complete and you can move to the next area requiring treatment.

## Treatment
### Don't forget the questions above for each reflex treated!

Hand-holds are given in detail in the assessment (Chapter Three) for treating the right foot reflex areas and should be reversed when treating the left foot.

*Solar plexus:* Massage the whole of this area with the side of the whole top half of your thumb in a circular motion as firmly as the tolerance of the individual person will allow, remembering your questions! If the client:

a) is highly stressed, even gentle stroking may seem painful.

b) is not stressed at all, there may be no reaction.

Whether the finding is a) or b), this reflex area should still be massaged.

Keep circling at the client's tolerance level, maintaining the same pressure throughout *(very important!)*, whilst continually asking if the 'pain' is easing a little. Keep circling – and asking – until the discomfort has completely gone.

If the reflex is still painful after one minute, the original pressure was obviously too strong and the movement should be repeated with just enough pressure for the person to feel moderate – not excruciating – pain at the start of the circling.

Remember to relax the pressure on the return half of every circle.

Repeat the solar plexus massage on the left foot.

*Problematic reflexes:* Using the order given in the assessment, massage (in circular movements as described above), only those reflex areas which presented a problem during the assessment technique.

This could be the spinal areas for backache or muscular aches and pains, etc.; the lung area if the client has bronchial problems; all digestive system areas for constipation (concentrating on the large intestine area) – and so on. Treat these troubled reflexes using the hand-holds given in the assessment technique, reversing them when treating the left foot.

*A reminder, should the digestive system need treating:*

1) Holding back the toes of the *right* foot with your right hand, massage the liver and gall bladder area with the ball of your left thumb.
2) Holding the *left* foot with your right hand, massage the stomach and small intestine areas with your left thumb.
3) Return to the *right* foot (holding it with your left hand) and massage the small intestine reflex area on that foot with your right thumb.
4) Passing through the ileocecal valve reflex, massage the ascending colon, followed by the first part of the transverse colon (still with your right thumb).
5) Returning once more to the *left* foot (holding it with the right hand), complete the treatment of the transverse colon.
6) Changing the hand-hold to your left hand, massage down the descending colon, then across the base of the colon to the anus with your right thumb.

(See pages 36-40)

*Excretory system:* When all the troubled areas have been covered, place your right hand over the person's right toes, taking them over to the left. With your left thumb, massage the kidney and ureter tube in an elongated circle, followed by circling the bladder reflex. Repeat on the other foot.

## Finishing massage

1) Wrapping one foot in a towel, apply a small amount of reflex cream over the whole of the foot.
2) With hands facing opposite ways but close together, place them behind one another with the palms on the top of the foot (4.1M). Take them up to the ankle, opening them as you get there, so that they are on either side of the foot (4.2M). Moving one hand underneath the foot and the other on top, return to the toes, sandwiching the foot very firmly in between your hands (4.3M). Repeat this sequence two or three times.
3) With fingers on top of the foot and thumbs overlapped (4.4M), take them from the centre to the outsides of the foot (4.5M), then back again. Zig-zag in this fashion down the sole of the foot from toes to heel then push very firmly all the way back to the toes (4.6M)
4) Holding the foot firmly with one hand, stroke firmly down the inner side of the sole with the palm of your other hand from ball of foot to heel (4.7M and 4.8M).
5) Wrap that foot in a towel to keep warm and apply a small amount of reflex cream to the other one.

   Repeat 2-5 on that foot, then wrap in a towel.

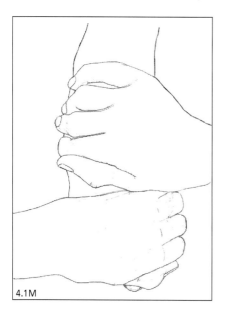

4.1M

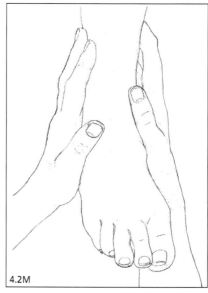

4.2M

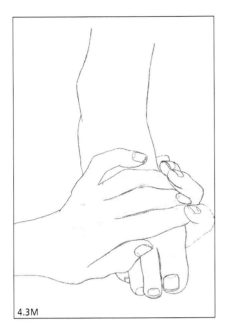

4.3M

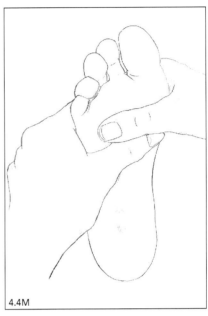

4.4M

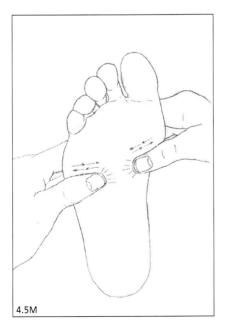

4.5M

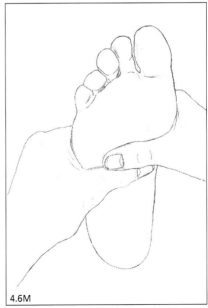

4.6M

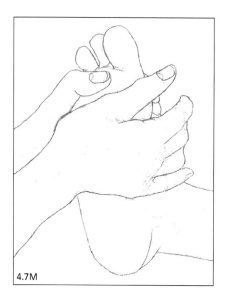

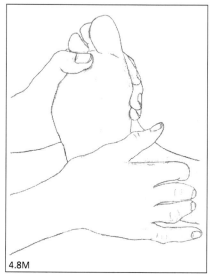

4.7M

4.8M

### Home Treatment

As the treatment should be done every day at home, either by the client's carer, friend or partner, for the best results to be achieved. That person should now change places with the therapist, who should guide the carer, friend or partner through the method of treatment, making sure it is done correctly.

*The location of reflex areas, and pressure applied, should be thoroughly checked.*

If the client will be doing self-treatments at home, he or she should be shown the technique by the therapist immediately after the treatment (Chapter Six).

- A diagram of the feet should be given to the client to take home, with the reflex areas to be massaged clearly marked and the order of work clearly numbered on those areas.
- An appointment should also be made for a second visit (again with carer, friend or partner), when the therapist should repeat the treatment, followed by watching the carer, friend or partner once more, to check that all is being done correctly.

I am emphasising these two points because, when a client of mine (who wore a surgical collar due to her neck problem) returned for her second treatment, disappointed that she felt no better, it came out that she had been massaging, not the neck of her big toe, but the soft cushion of the big toe itself (the pituitary gland reflex!). After that, she began showing improvement, eventually doing away with her surgical collar (see page 84). This experience emphasises the importance of giving clients a marked chart, showing exactly the position of the reflex points to be massaged, as well as the sequence of the treatment.

Finally, as the client will be given the reflex cream used in the treatment to take home, he/she should be asked not to forget to bring it back for the follow-up treatment!

# Chapter Five
# Aromaflexology for Babies

Aromaflexology is a very simple and effective way of helping babies through their minor ailments, especially those concerning digestion. It is not necessary to know where the individual reflex points are as, because a baby's feet are very small and the whole centre of the soles of his* feet will be treated.

Babies and children, being smaller, will obviously need a lower concentration of essential oils than adults, with the concentration for babies being even lower than that of children.

### Why is baby crying?
It is not always easy to decide what is causing discomfort in a baby. Does he need a clean nappy, or a feed? Or is he suffering from wind, toothache, nausea, colic, constipation or stomach pain? All baby can do to tell you something is wrong is to cry!

Nappies can be checked, as can the last time a feed was given, but for the rest, it is mainly guesswork. This is where aromaflexology can be such a help to a worried mother.

There are no reflex points or special hand-holds to learn for treatment of a baby, as the whole sole of the foot can be massaged, covering the solar plexus and all the digestive system with each circular movement; the treatment will therefore benefit most presenting conditions affecting the baby's digestive and nervous systems.

### Essential oils to use
Many essential oils are beneficial for babies but most should be administered by a qualified aromatherapist; however, the four oils below are safe for parents to use and are also useful for the most common ailments affecting babies. These are:

• Roman chamomile [*Chamaemelum nobile*] – aids sleep; relieves infantile diarrhoea, wind, indigestion and colic; calming; reduces pain and gum inflammation when teething (for the latter, the big toe cushions should be massaged).

* (For ease, baby will be referred to as 'him' throughout.)

• lavender [*Lavandula angustifolia*] – aids sleep; relieves colic and wind; calming and soothing
• sweet orange [*Citrus sinensis*] – aids sleep; calming; normalising effect on both constipation and diarrhoea; relieves both indigestion and wind
• peppermint [*Mentha* x *piperita*] – ideal for colic, indigestion and wind

As can be seen from the above:
All four essential oils relieve trapped wind – so often experienced by babies!
The first three are excellent for helping baby to sleep; if baby is not sleeping well, giving an aromaflexology treatment before bed will help to settle him down.
The same three are also calming, so giving baby a treatment if he seems overactive, stressed or crying for no apparent reason would help to quieten him.
Roman chamomile and lavender are both analgesic, so can help baby when he is in pain.
Roman chamomile, lavender and peppermint help to overcome colic, which is also quite common in babies.
Roman chamomile and peppermint both relieve indigestion.

As only 3-4 essential oils are needed to treat most of baby's ailments, only one cream containing these is necessary to help all of them.

**Mixing the cream**
As the percentage of essential oil in the cream has to be much less than that for an adult, baby's cream should be made up as follows:

• 30 ml base cream
• 3 drops each of Roman chamomile, lavender and sweet orange
• 2 drops of peppermint oil

Peppermint essential oil is excellent for digestive problems. However, as it has a powerful aroma, two drops in the 30 ml of base cream is sufficient to help relieve symptoms.
N.B. Peppermint oil should not be added if baby is breastfed, as it is anti-lactogenic (it can hinder the secretion of milk).

**Method of work**
New parents have no difficulty touching, stroking and cuddling their babies and it is a very small step from there to giving them an aromaflexology treatment to ease any discomfort they may be suffering.

For contact to be made easily and comfortably with baby's feet, sit along the length of a sofa, supporting your back on cushions or pillows (Price & Price 2009). Placing a warm soft towel over your tummy, lay your baby on it (on his back, head facing away from you), drawing your knees towards you to support him.

1) Put a very small amount of cream on baby's right foot and lower leg. Holding his foot with your right hand, massage his lower leg briefly and gently with your left hand.
2) Gently hold baby's ankle between your right-hand fingers and with as much of the length of your thumb as possible move in slow circles over the centre of the sole of his foot, for about half a minute (see diagram below).
3) Repeat movement 1.
4) Apply a very small amount of cream on baby's left foot and lower leg and repeat movements 1-3, remembering to change hands.

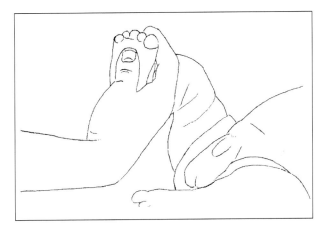

Not only will baby benefit from his aromaflexology experience and both mother and baby enjoy it, but it will help reduce any stress the mother may be feeling.

**Reference**
*Aromatherapy for Babies and Children*. Price S; Price P. 2009 Riverhead.

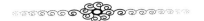

Aromaflexology

# Chapter Six
# Self-Treatment

Aromaflexologists can, like anyone else, succumb to a health problem and may wish to ameliorate it by using aromaflexology. As it may be difficult for them to find an aromaflexologist in their area, this chapter enables them to treat themselves with the success they love having with their clients – I have often treated myself with positive results – see page 79, for one of them.

Not only aromaflexologists, but whoever does the client's daily treatments (carer, family member or friend) may possibly appreciate being able to help themselves, and although it would be preferable for them to see a qualified aromaflexologist, if they have only a simple health problem, this chapter is ideal if they would like to try to help themselves by using aromaflexology.

As these people have given a client his or her daily treatment at home, they are well versed in the position of the reflexes. Having watched a professional at work and been shown exactly what to do, followed then by doing it on the client under guidance of the therapist, it is possible for them also, with the help of this chapter, to carry out a self-treatment.

When treating oneself, although the same order of work is followed, the hand-holds and method of work are often slightly different. For example, in the spine, one can massage upwards towards the big toe if this is found easier, instead of downwards towards the heel, as when treating someone else.

Most people have an idea of what they are suffering from; however, do not hesitate to give yourself an assessment, or go and see your GP, if you are not sure of the reason for your condition.

Some reflexes are easier to treat on oneself than others – for example, the spine is easy to reach, but the hip and knee reflexes are quite difficult to find as they are located on the outside edge of the foot. Nevertheless, it can be done with the help of a chair on either side of you.

Having decided which reflexes you are going to treat, select your essential oils –
by the same method described in Chapter Four, then mix the cream. Sit comfortably
on a chair, with a second chair (kitchen or dining) at each side of you.

Always start your treatment with the solar plexus reflexes, to make sure you are
relaxed, and finish with the excretory system, to help any toxins to be drained into the
bladder and excreted.

## Nervous system

**Solar plexus:** Firstly, place your right foot across your left knee and, supporting
it around the ankle with your right hand, do circles on the solar plexus area with
your left thumb up to your own pain threshold. Circle at this pressure until the
pain completely disappears. The maximum time to work on one reflex at any one
treatment is two minutes – even on yourself.

Replace this foot with your left one, holding it with your left hand and repeat the
circles on the solar plexus reflex with your right thumb. Continue by treating only the
reflexes representing an imbalance in your body. Treat a complete system on each
foot before changing to the next system.

**Sciatic nerve:** To treat the sciatic nerve, place your right foot across your left knee,
supporting it as before. With your left thumb, do circles on the sole of your foot along the
top edge of the heel cushion, then, using your middle finger, do elongated circles on the
outside edge of the foot, from the top of the heel cushion to the base of the heel (along
the bony part).

Replace this foot with your left one, reversing the hand-hold and repeating the
circles with your right thumb and middle finger.

## Glandular system (*pituitary, parathyroid, thyroid*)
## Sinuses, eyes and ears

These reflexes are easy to find and treat, using the same principles as for the solar
plexus reflex above.

## Bone and muscular system

**Spine:** Place your right foot across your left knee and supporting it around the ankle
with your right hand, do elongated circles with your left hand, either from the base of
the big toe to just above the waist level, or from the waist towards your big toe, if that
proves easier. Move to the level of the kidney reflex and repeat the circling between
there and the waist of your foot.

Now circle from the bottom edge of the heel up the bony part as far as your
bladder reflex – without actually touching it.

**Neck:** Using your left thumb, circle in each part of the neck reflex.

**Shoulders:** use your left thumb for this reflex.

*Elbow:* move your right hand to pull the toes towards you. Use your left middle finger to treat the elbow reflex.

*Hip:* With your middle finger "glued" to the hip reflex point do on-the-spot circles. If you find it difficult to reach the reflex, you may find it easier and more comfortable to put your foot on the nearest chair to it, and massage the reflex with your thumb cushion.

*Knee:* Technique as for the hip.

Place your left foot across your right knee to repeat the treatment of the whole muscular system.

## Respiratory system

*Lungs:* Place your right foot across your left knee and, supporting it round the ankle with your right hand, do two elongated circles on the ball of the foot with your left hand, from the diaphragm nearly up to the toes, doing the first row of circles between the third and fourth toe and the second row between the second and third toes.

Placing your left foot across your right knee repeat the respiratory treatment on this foot, using your right thumb for the circles.

## Digestive system

To treat this system, it is necessary to go from one foot to the other and back again in order to cover the digestive organs in sequence:

*Liver:* Place the right foot over the left knee and supporting the foot with your right hand, do circles with your left thumb over the liver reflex area.

*Gall bladder:* Keeping the same hold, circle over the gall bladder reflex.

*Pancreas:* Place the left foot over the right knee and support it with your left hand.

The pancreas reflex overlaps the lower edge of the stomach – so bear this in mind in mind if an unpleasant reaction is obtained whilst doing this reflex. Try to keep as near to the inside edge of the foot as you can, to try and avoid a crossover with the stomach reflex

*Stomach:* Keeping the same hold, circle with your right thumb over the uppermost part of the stomach reflex area, thus avoiding that covered whilst doing the pancreas.

*Small intestine:* Keeping the same hold, take your thumb just below the waist of your foot to the small intestine reflex area and carry out the circling technique there.

Changing feet, hold the right foot with your left hand and repeat the circling on the rest of the small intestine reflex with your right thumb.

*Large intestine:* Still using your right thumb, slide over the ileocaecal valve, and do elongated circles up the ascending colon with your right thumb, continuing across the transverse colon reflex to the inner side of your foot.

Changing feet once again (holding the left foot with your right hand), continue the elongated circles, using your left thumb, across the rest of the transverse colon reflex, down the descending colon, finishing across the base of the colon to the anus.

## Reproductive system

**Ovaries:** Place your right leg over your left knee, holding the outside of the foot with your right hand. Taking your left hand over your right arm, circle the ovary reflex (outside edge of foot) with your middle finger.

**Fallopian tube:** Caterpillar with pressure (still using your left middle finger) up the fallopian tube as far as you can, then, bringing your foot towards you, caterpillar the rest of the way to the uterus reflex with your right thumb.

**Uterus:** Gently circle the uterus reflex with your right thumb.

Reverse hand-holds to treat the left foot, right arm over left this time, to circle the ovary reflex with your right middle finger and the uterus with your right thumb.

## Circulatory system

**Heart:** If you have a heart condition, the area of the heart reflex may be treated – very gently. Place your left foot over your right knee and, holding the toes with your left hand, circle the heart area gently for one minute.

**Cervical lymph:** Keeping your left foot over your right knee, support it at the ankle with your left hand. Move your right thumb slowly with pressure (on the top of the foot) between the first and second toes and second and third toes, from the toes downwards for about an inch, repeating as necessary till any pain felt is gone.

**Groin lymph:** Keeping the same hold, circle with pressure at the end of the fallopian tube, just above the uterus.

Repeat on right foot, changing feet and hand-holds.

## Excretory system

**Kidney and ureter tube:** Place the left foot over the right knee, holding the toes firmly with the left hand. Using your right thumb and starting on the kidney reflex, push firmly down the ureter tube reflex to the bladder, returning lightly. Repeat these elongated circles as long as is necessary.

**Bladder:** Keeping the same hold, do pressured circles on the bladder reflex.

Repeat on right foot, changing feet and hand-holds.

Each day, after the treatment, apply a little of your cream over both feet, especially round your heels; this will keep your skin soft and prevent hard skin forming on your heels.

I have done aromaflexology on myself for years, whenever I have had a health problem, with considerable success for most of them. I do it whilst watching television in the evening, as I have so many other things to see to during the day. The main thing is to have a set time, so that one is less likely to forget!

The first time I needed to treat myself is recounted in Case Study 6 on page 79, when my reflex cream was made with essential oils to help to relax muscles. To save having several reflex creams in my cupboard, when I need a treatment for something different, I simply add a couple of oils to the existing cream (having checked first if any of the original ones would help my second problem). As I rarely have a health concern and most of my needs have been muscular (ie a new hip twice), the cream has lasted me for several years – essential oils do not have a shelf life, except maybe 4000 years – think of the entombed Pharaohs!

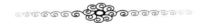

# Chapter Seven
# Shoulder Massage

B efore I retired, whenever a member of our staff had a headache, neck pain, or was stressed about something, I used to carry out the following massage with great success. Within minutes, the member of staff felt well enough to return to his or her work. I always finished aromaflexology treatments with this shoulder massage, ensuring clients were completely relaxed before driving home.

## Introduction

### General massage

Although a qualification is required to give a professional body massage, clients can still benefit from caring touch given by an inexperienced or non-qualified person. The intention of the treatment given is the same – to relieve both muscular and nervous tension. Nothing can replace hands-on, whether or not the person giving the massage is qualified – the important thing is that the therapist should devote complete attention to the client and not be thinking of other things whilst giving the massage.

Knowledge of a few simple techniques, such as those described in this chapter, is an extremely valuable asset which can bring relief and comfort to the person on the receiving end and when essential oils are blended into the massage medium, not only are the benefits enhanced, but the effects are longer lasting.

The word massage originally comes from the Arabic word 'massa', meaning to touch, feel or handle and is one of the oldest forms of treatment for human ailments. Hippocrates (460 to 380 BC) said about a dislocated shoulder – "it is necessary to rub the shoulder gently and smoothly with soft hands. The physician must be experienced in many things, but surely also in rubbing". Since then various systems and techniques have been developed over the centuries.

**67**

Through massage all the functions of the bodily organs – skin, muscles, nerves, glands, etc – are stimulated, and by the increased circulation of the blood and lymph the clearing away of body waste is assisted. Furthermore, massage and its effects are always enhanced by the use of essential oils, which are an additional aid to reducing tension, whether in the back, legs or upper neck and shoulder area. The movements can vary from soft, light, rhythmical stroking movements designed to relax the muscles and nerves, to kneading, which is designed to break up tension nodules. Where a client is suffering from general stress, it is a good idea to give a shoulder massage after the aromaflexology treatment, as this helps to reduce their stress still further.

### Essential oils used

The massage oil should be made up of 5 ml of sunflower seed or other light vegetable oil, to which has been added 6-8 drops of stress-reducing essential oils which may already be in the client's reflex cream. If there are none in the cream, add 6-8 drops of any stress-reducing oils of your choice (see p. 94).

To apply it, put a little into the palm of one hand, then rub both hands together lightly, to distribute the oil evenly.

## Massage techniques

### Effleurage

This is a stroking movement, always done using the whole hand, with emphasis on the palm. The hands should be relaxed and mould themselves to the part of the body being massaged. They should keep contact with the body all the time and the rhythm of the strokes should be slow and even.

Effleurage improves the venous flow – it helps to remove congestion in the veins, so that fresh blood can circulate more freely, taking nutrients to all organs through which it passes. As an added bonus, it is extremely soothing and relaxing, particularly for nervous, irritated or over-tired people.

Two types of stroking are used in massage:

- deep stroking - done with the whole hand with pressure, and always in the direction of the heart, which helps the venous flow.
- superficial stroking, also done with the whole hand but in the return direction from deep stroking and *without* pressure.

### Frictions

Frictions are little circles, usually carried out with pressure, using the cushions of the thumbs or one or more fingers, and are excellent for breaking down tension nodules. After several circles over one area have been completed, the pressure is released so that the hand (*without losing contact*) can slide to the next area and the movement repeated.

**68**

Pressure must be firm but not such as to cause injury to the underlying tissues.

Frictions aid the removal of excess fluid in the body and stimulate circulation. It is important for massage movements to be done correctly and the best results are obviously obtained by visiting a qualified masseur. However, as in all arts, such as cooking, painting, pottery, etc, many people, without professional training, possess a natural ability to carry out these arts, and with a little help (to make sure their technique is correct) these people can reach a good standard.

### *Kneading*

Kneading is when a muscle, or part of a muscle group, is picked up, squeezed and released while the other hand moves to the adjacent area to repeat the process. Kneading usually requires both hands, using the palm, the fingers or the thumbs, depending on the size of the muscle area being massaged.

It is essential that this movement is carried out only after the area has been previously relaxed by effleurage, and it should be slow, gentle and rhythmical, always returning to the starting point with a superficial stroke, without a break in contact.

Kneading also increases circulation and helps the removal of waste products.

As a general rule the tensions and anxieties we feel show themselves first of all as nodules in the shoulder muscles and/or neck. It is not always apparent as pain, though this can be felt immediately if someone presses firmly on the exact area of these tight muscle fibres, which are called nodules.

Shoulder and neck massage is best done with the client sitting straddled on a low backed chair - facing the chair back and resting the arms and head on a cushion which has been placed on the chair back.

The following sequence can be used to relieve headaches and shoulder tension and will also promote general relaxation. Using frictions over hard tension nodules in the shoulder and neck helps to relax tight muscles, which stimulates a general release of tension throughout the body.

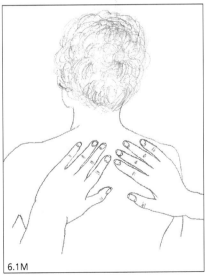

6.1M

## Shoulder and neck massage

1) Stand behind your client with one foot pointing forward and the other at right angles to it, and slightly behind.
   Make sure your hands are relaxed before placing them gently at the base of each shoulder blade (6.1M).

Begin with effleurage, using both hands (with spaces between your relaxed fingers), applying firm pressure from the bottom of the shoulder blades up each side of the spine up to the base of the neck (the pressure should be equal on both fingers and palms of both hands).

The movement is continued by moving your hands apart across the top of the shoulders, cradling the shoulders with the whole of each hand, then bringing them lightly round and down to the starting point.

Repeat this several times, finishing with a light return stroke.

2) With your fingers at the base of each shoulder blade, do friction movements in the spinal channel with your thumbs, up either side of the spine, (6.2M), taking the whole of both relaxed hands across the shoulders and lightly back to the starting point. Repeat several times.

3) a. Without removing your hands from the client, walk around to the left-hand side of the chair, so that your client's left shoulder is directly facing the centre of your body. Your feet should be about 45 cm apart, so that you can bend your knees; this will enable you to carry out the movements effectively without strain.

3) b. Place your left hand (in an L shape with your thumb and your fingers) over your client's shoulder – thumb behind the shoulder (6.3M).

Using firm pressure, move your hand slowly up to the neck, swinging your body to the right as you bend your right knee.

When the left hand almost reaches the hairline, swing your body over to the left as you bend your left knee, so that your right hand (also L-shaped) can follow smoothly behind the left one.

Now lift off your left hand, and as the right hand almost reaches the neck, swing your body over to the right again, enabling you to bring in the left hand once more (6.4M).

Lift off the right hand and, maintaining a good rhythm, repeat the sequence with alternate hands for several seconds.

4) With your thumbs, feel for painful tension nodules in the top shoulder area. Where these occur, use the cushion of alternate thumbs in firm short strokes over the area (6.5M).

For very hard nodules, use firm pressure with only one thumb, replacing it with the other one if the first becomes tired.

Apply sufficient pressure to reach your client's pain threshold, but take care not to go beyond it.

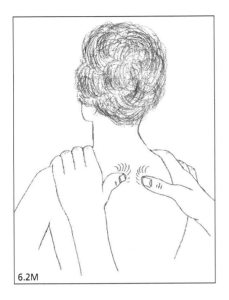

6.2M

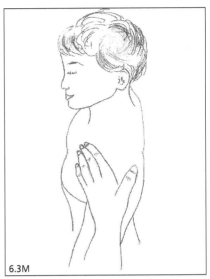

6.3M

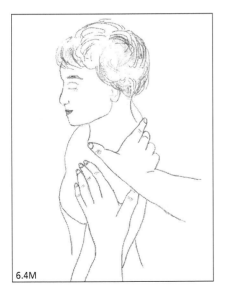

6.4M

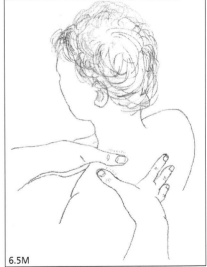

6.5M

Circle firmly with your thumbs for several seconds over all nodules requiring softening.

5) Without altering your stance, repeat movements 6.3M and 6.4M.

6) Keeping your right hand in contact with the shoulder, place your left hand gently across the client's forehead. Make a 'V' with your right hand at the centre base of the back of the neck and move it up to the hairline slowly, with pressure, gently squeezing as you go (6.6M). Return to the base of the neck with a light stroke and repeat several times.

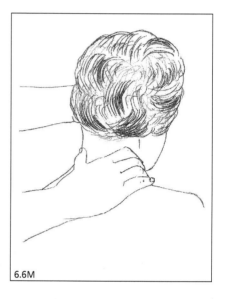

6.6M

7) Keeping one hand in contact with the client, walk round the chair to the right shoulder and repeat movements 3 – 6. NB Remember you are now working on the right shoulder, so will be starting 3b with the *right* hand, not the left.

8) Still with your hands in contact with the body, walk behind your client and repeat movement 1, gradually ending gently with your fingertips at the centre base of the shoulders and lightly lifting them off.

The client's shoulders should not be greasy after the massage is finished. If they are, it is because too much oil has been used and the shoulders should be wiped with a soft paper towel before the client gets dressed.

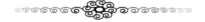

# Chapter Eight
# Case Histories

The following cases were chosen from many carried out by aromatherapists trained in aromaflexology by myself, my daughter and those qualified from other aromatherapy schools teaching the subject. Aromatherapists without this training may have good results if the instructions in this book are carried out to the letter ; – but – training at a college is the best answer!

**Bronchial Asthma** (Shirley Price). **Constipation** (Debbie Moore). **Constipation and Thyroid** (Lora Cantele). **Insomnia and Constipation** (Lora Cantele). **Indigestion and Insomnia** (Lora Cantele). **Muscular – Back** [self-treatment] (Shirley Price). **Muscular – Back** (Karen Green). **Severe Sinusitis** (Shirley Price). **Spinal problems: Crumbling Vertebrae; Mining Accident; Severe Neck Problem; Whiplash** (Shirley Price). **Stress and Diarrhoea** (Lora Cantele*)*. **Stress with Muscular Tension** (Shirley Price*)*. **Stress, Shoulder Pain and Plantar Fasciitis** (Karen Green).

## 1. Bronchial Asthma

### *Assessment*
My husband Len's asthma was the first ailment I tried to help after completing my course on reflexology with Doreen Bayley. He has two inhalers and was using them quite frequently.

His breathing problems accelerate in certain conditions i.e. when it is very cold he cannot be outside for long before breathing becomes difficult. He's also allergic to certain perfumes and has often been moved to first class on an aeroplane if sitting next to a lady who has been testing perfumes in the duty-free shop – they never let me go with him!

However, he is *never* allergic to essential oils – perfume only affects him because many ingredients are synthetic; synthetics are stable and necessarily have a much longer lasting aroma than essential oils, which are absorbed into the bloodstream and whose composition varies each year, depending on soil and weather conditions.

### Treatment

When I decided to replace reflexology with that of aromaflexology, I made up a jar of the following essential oils in 30 ml of a bland base cream:

- 10 drops peppermint [*Mentha x piperita*] – antiinflammatory, expectorant, hypotensor
- 10 drops Tasmanian blue gum [*Eucalyptus globulus*] – anticatarrhal, antiinfectious, antiinflammatory, decongestant, mucolytic
- 5 drops hyssop [*Hyssopus officinalis*] – anticatarrhal, antiinflammatory, mucolytic
- 5 drops sage [*Salvia officinalis*] – anticatarrhal, expectorant, hypotensor, mucolytic

Many aromatherapists are unnecessarily afraid to use hyssop. For someone with limited knowledge I would agree (a *little* knowledge can be a dangerous thing), but a properly qualified aromatherapist should never fear of using essential oils with powerful components; these are frequently needed to enhance the beneficial effect, provided they are used with intelligence and in the correct dilution.

As stated in Chapter Four, so little cream is applied at any one aromaflexology treatment, that 30 drops of essential oils in 30 ml of the base cream is not too strong. I gave him a treatment every day, starting with the solar plexus reflex, followed by the lung area and finishing with the kidney/bladder area to help any toxins to be eliminated.

### Outcome

Gradually, over a period of about three months, he was able to do without his inhalers, except for emergencies. He now only needs them if he meets someone with a perfume to which he is allergic (fortunately, he is not allergic to all synthetics) or gets into a lift which has just been cleaned with a product containing artificial aromas. I no longer need to give him aromaflexology treatments regularly. Whenever he is affected suddenly by anything which makes breathing difficult, he puts a bottle containing a mix of the pure essential oils above against his finger, then places the latter on the base of his nostrils. If suffering simply from a blocked nose, he puts 4 to 6 drops onto a tissue and inhales deeply three times to clear it.

A few years ago Len had to go out of church on days when incense was used. Recently, the church changed the frankincense used, as they discovered that other people were affected too; they now buy their incense from a supplier who uses natural products.

## 2. Constipation

### Assessment

Jane brought her 8-year-old son Robert to see me – he was suffering with constipation, only evacuating his bowels once or twice a week.

Robert had Spinal Muscular Atrophy, where the link between the nerves and muscles breaks down. This affected his legs, causing curvature of the spine. Due to the lack of mobility in his lower body his digestion was sluggish. The constipation made him feel uncomfortable and miserable, which greatly concerned his Mum. After discussing the problem, I decided to offer Robert an aromaflexology treatment.

On assessing the reflex points on his feet it was indeed evident that the colon was very congested as the reflex was very uncomfortable on touching.

### Treatment

A base cream was made up containing essential oils of:

- sweet marjoram [*Origanum majorana*] – analgesic, antispasmodic, calming, digestive, neurotonic
- sweet orange [*Citrus sinensis*] – antidepressant, antispasmodic, calming, stomachic
- ginger [*Zingiber officinale*] – analgesic, digestive

I proceeded to massage his small feet, covering the solar plexus, the digestive reflexes, especially the colon, finishing with the kidney area to clear the toxins. The colon was very sensitive but Robert and I persevered and I managed to spend about 5 – 7 minutes on each foot. We had a lovely conversation throughout the treatment and I showed Jane how to massage Robert's feet, so that she could do it every night, to help still further with his digestion and clear the colon. Robert and Jane left feeling very confident with the information that I had given them.

### Outcome

The wonderful outcome of this treatment is that Jane contacted me several days afterwards to inform me that Robert had been to the toilet and cleared his bowels two days running! She was ecstatic, because her little boy's mood had improved along with his bowel movements! She maintained the daily routine until Robert's bowels had settled into a regular pattern.

## 3. Constipation and Thyroid

### Assessment
Ms. F, a 39-year-old, complained of a thyroid malfunction, sluggish bowel, weight gain and high cholesterol. She exercised (Jazzercise, cycling, weightlifting) at least 3 times per week, but admitted to heavy consumption of white bread and potatoes and a late night snack of cookies or ice cream. She is not on medication but takes a multivitamin (infrequently) and a herbal remedy (iodine) for thyroid concerns. Discomfort showed in the thyroid, lymph and renal reflex areas and during her assessment, she said her stool varied from "very loose" to "complete constipation".

### Treatment
The following essential oils were added to 1 oz./30 ml of bland white cream:

- 10 drops Roman chamomile [*Chamaemelum nobile*] – antispasmodic; calming; digestive
- 8 drops ginger [*Zingiber officinale*] – analgesic; digestive
- 4 drops clove bud [*Syzygium aromaticum*] – hormone-like
- 4 drops geranium [*Pelargonium graveolens*] – astringent; decongestant (lymph); digestive
- 4 drops juniper branch [*Juniperus communis ram.*] – depurative (digestive system and kidneys)

The treatment was carried out on her solar plexus, neck, thyroid and lymph, followed by the digestive system and finishing with the renal reflexes. Ms. F was then shown how to carry out the massage on herself, to do at home each night before bed. She was also given some dietary advice and asked to return in a week for a follow-up.

### Outcome
At her second appointment I found she had carried out her aromaflexology with the correct technique. She reported some improvement in her health, especially with regard to her stools. It was recommended that she continue self-care at home.

A phone call replaced the next follow-up visit in which Ms. F indicated she was feeling in much better health and less stressed, despite her busy work schedule. Her stools appeared to have normalized also.

## 4. Insomnia and Constipation

### Assessment
Judy (not her real name) is 39 and suffers from restless sleep, constipation, neck and shoulder pain and low energy. She has a fairly nutritious diet and drinks plenty of water, leaving caffeine and snacks alone. She exercises daily.

### Treatment

30 drops of the following essential oils were blended in 1 oz/30 ml of base cream:

- 10 drops lavender [*Lavandula angustifolia*] – analgesic; calming/sedative; tonic
- 8 drops mandarin [*Citrus reticulata*] – calming; digestive
- 7 drops bitter orange [*Citrus aurantium* var. *amara* per.] – digestive; sedative
- 5 drops rosemary [*Rosmarinus officinalis*] – analgesic; digestive

A very small amount of the blend was massaged into those reflexes which had given discomfort in the assessment.

After the treatment, Judy was shown how to carry out her own reflex massage on the affected areas – and asked to do this daily.

### Outcome

Judy returned for a follow-up visit after 11 days. She presented at this session with the addition of anxiety, saying that her economic situation had drastically changed as she had just lost her job.

There was slight improvement in her digestive complaints, but her stress was evident by the reaction on her solar plexus.

The following oils were added to her cream, giving more emphasis to her nervous system and constipation. She was also asked to give herself the treatment twice daily instead of once.

- 8 drops sweet marjoram [*Origanum majorana*] – analgesic; calming; neurotonic
- 6 drops basil [*Ocimum basilicum*] – analgesic; calming; digestive; neurotonic

### Final Outcome

I followed up with Judy two weeks later. She had been performing her aromaflexology massage twice each day and it had greatly helped her sleep quality and her anxiety.

10 days later she reported that she was sleeping better, suffering less from constipation and her shoulder pain was very much improved.

## 5. Indigestion and Insomnia

### Assessment

Client K is a 37-year-old woman who is an admitted workaholic. Her occupation is training executives and teams in the areas of Leadership, Business Development, and Time Management.

K is an avid runner and runs daily. She is in good general health; a non-smoker, moderate drinker and she eats nutritious meals (when not travelling).

K came to my office seeking relief from gastrointestinal upset. She was affected by nagging discomfort in her stomach and painful indigestion when she ate. During the assessment she also disclosed that she was having difficulty falling and staying asleep. Thus the three dominant needs to be addressed were stress, insomnia and digestion.

### Treatment
The following essential oils were prepared in 1 oz/30 ml bland natural white cream:

- 8 drops lemon [*Citrus limon*] – digestive (painful); calming
- 8 drops sweet marjoram [*Origanum majorana*] – calming (anxiety, insomnia); digestive
- 5 drops rose [*Rosa damascena*] – anxiety, stress
- 4 drops ylang ylang [*Cananga odorata*] – calming, sedative
- 3 drops sandalwood [*Santalum album*] – sedative
- 2 drops vetiver [*Vetiveria zizanoides*] – immunostimulant

After giving K an aromaflexology massage I asked her to follow through at home each evening with the self-treatment technique I had shown her, using the cream I had blended.

### Outcome
On checking K when she returned five days later, I found she was doing her self-treatment correctly. She said she'd been sleeping much better and that while her job wasn't any less stressful, she believed her self-care was helping her manage it better. She also said her digestive issue had seemed to improve somewhat.

When she came for her next visit ten days later she said she was sleeping well and felt less stressed; she also no longer had indigestion, remarking that the "digestive oils" I had selected must have done the trick!

I saw K several months later, when she told me that she credits aromaflexology for her healing - she now uses the cream as a nightly "foot cream", rather than focusing on the reflexes.

### Reference
Price S and Price L. (2007 – 3rd edition). *Aromatherapy for Health Professionals*. London: Churchill Livingstone.

## 6. Muscular – Back (self-treatment)

### *Assessment*

Several years ago I was asked to open the shop of a customer of ours in Blackpool. Just before leaving the house, I turned quickly whilst sitting down – and my back 'went'. It was agony – I couldn't move and Len wanted to ring the shop to cancel. I couldn't let them down, so I persuaded him to carry me to the car – and we set off.

### *Treatment*

All the way there (a 2½ hour journey) I did aromaflexology (called Swiss Reflex Treatment then) on my spinal reflexes, using my base cream with the following essential oils, pausing only to rest my thumbs from time to time:

- 10 drops Tasmanian blue gum [*Eucalyptus globulus*] – antiinflammatory, rubefacient
- 10 drops rosemary [*Rosmarinus officinalis*] – analgesic, antiinflammatory, neuromuscular
- 4 drops sweet marjoram [*Origanum majorana*] – analgesic, antiinflammatory, antispasmodic
- 8 drops lavender [*Lavandula angustifolia*] – analgesic, antiinflammatory, antispasmodic

### *Outcome:*

When we arrived at the shop, Len helped me out of the car – and I was able to walk (albeit slowly) into the shop, and give my opening speech – success!

## 7. Muscular – Back

### *Assessment*

G. Mounac presented with severe back pain for which he was being treated in Toulouse Hospital back pain clinic and was currently on morphine to cope with the pain. Due to the severity of the back pain, it was decided that aromaflexology was preferable to back massage.

### *Treatment*

As the client was also stressed through being in constant pain, the choice of oils was as follows:

- Roman chamomile [*Chamaemelum nobile*] – antiinflammatory, antispasmodic, calming/sedative

- lavender [*Lavandula angustifolia*] – analgesic, antiinflammatory, calming/sedative; tonic
- sweet marjoram [*Origanum majorana*] – analgesic, antispasmodic, calming, neurotonic

### Outcome

Gilles came each week for six weeks. On the second visit, he had noticed a difference and was not in so much pain for a day or so. He and his partner had been shown which areas to massage at home daily to maximise the effects and on the third visit he said the time without pain had not only increased, but he had actually come off the morphine patches.

He was advised to continue using aromaflexology at home on an ongoing basis between each visit and return for a check-up in two months' time. He told me he was very grateful for the improvement it had made and that he and his partner were going to continue doing aromaflexology at home.

## 8. Severe Sinusitis

### Assessment

Peter's wife had heard me on the radio and although she and her husband lived over 60 miles away, he wanted to come and see me. He had had chronic sinusitis for years and his sense of smell had deteriorated over time – he was suffering from prolonged temporary anosmia.

After an operation there was no improvement and he found life without being able to smell made him quite miserable at times, especially on his return from work, when he couldn't smell the dinner his wife had cooked for him (she was an excellent cook too!). Worse – he couldn't taste it either, as smell and taste are very closely linked. The problem was causing him a considerable amount of stress too, which affected his work.

### Treatment

I gave him a "sandwich" treatment – facial massage, concentrating on the sinus pressure points, followed by aromaflexology on the solar plexus reflex (for longer than the normal time at a treatment), then the sinus reflexes, finishing with the urinary system reflexes. I then completed the sandwich by repeating the facial treatment.

In the synergistic mix I included two very powerful essential oils to help his sinusitis (peppermint and eucalyptus), although he could not detect either of them. Included in the blend were two oils to relieve his stress:

- peppermint [*Mentha x piperita*] – analgesic, antiinflammatory, neurotonic
- Tasmanian blue gum [*Eucalyptus globulus*]– antiinfectious, antiinflammatory, mucolytic

- lavender [*Lavandula officinalis*] – antiseptic, balancing, calming
- sweet marjoram [*Origanum majorana*] – antiinfectious, calming, neurotonic

He didn't want to do aromaflexology on himself, but was more than willing to do the hour long journey every week and also to take home a bottle of the neat essential oils to inhale every night and three times during the day (using three *deep* breaths each time). I also gave him a lotion containing the essential oils above and taught him how to do the sinus pressure points on his face – to be done twice a day (which he was *quite* happy to do!).

### *Outcome*

He came every Saturday for a treatment and during the third visit, he suddenly said – "I think I can smell something!" I immediately put some peppermint onto a spill and held it up to his nose. He let out a delighted yell and said "I can smell mint! – it's *very* faint, but I *can* smell it!"

His sense of smell continued to improve and after six months he had recovered it sufficiently to be able to appreciate the aromas from his wife's cooking – which made life happier for both of them.

I had hoped he would have *some* results, however small, but in fact they were far better than I expected – with the unexpected side effect of making their marriage happier!

NB: I had just read about some recent findings by Wysocki *et al* (van Toller and Dodd 1992), which indicated that in man and animals presenting specific anosmia, the sensitivity to some odours can be restored by repeated exposure to these odours. The article was entitled 'Individual sufferances in olfactory ability'.

### *Reference*

Van Toller S, Dodd GH 1992 Fragrance: *The Psychology and Biology of Perfume*. Elsevier, London: 99-101

## 9. Spinal – Crumbling Vertebrae

### *Assessment*

My neighbour in France recommended one of her friends to come to me. Because M. Lesieur's discs between his vertebrae were crumbling, his specialist had told him he would have to have his vertebrae pinned together. He was suffering a lot of pain, was having difficulty in walking and wasn't sleeping at all well.

I told my neighbour that I probably wouldn't be able to help him at all but she said "Well, you'll have to see him now because he's coming tomorrow afternoon"!

M. Lesieur arrived the next day with his wife and it took him a full four minutes to walk from the car to our door. I knew straight away that an aromatherapy massage would be pointless, so I explained that aromaflexology may be able to help, but that they shouldn't expect any miracles.

He told me his one wish was to be able to decorate his house again and do odd jobs; he loved painting, papering and doing odd jobs in the house, but could no longer climb a ladder.

### Treatment

The oils selected for M. Lesieur, in 30 ml of bland reflex cream base were:

- lemon scented gum [*Eucalyptus citriodora*] – analgesic, antiinflammatory, calming
- juniper branch [*Juniperus communis ram.*] – analgesic, antiinflammatory, neurotonic
- frankincense [*Boswellia carteri*] – analgesic, antidepressive, antiinflammatory, immunostimulant
- lavender [*Lavandula angustifolia*] – analgesic, antiinflammatory, soporific, general tonic

I treated his solar plexus, neck and spine reflexes, finishing with the kidney/bladder reflexes. After I had finished, I taught his wife how to do these reflexes on her husband and she was very interested to learn.

I decided to give him a shoulder massage too, which I felt would help him to sleep, and along with the reflex cream, gave him some pure essential oils to inhale every night half an hour before going to bed.

I asked them to return four days later so that I could check his wife was massaging the reflexes correctly. She was incredibly good, as good as – or better – than some of the students I had taught!

### Outcome

M. Lesieur told me on arrival that he had slept ever since his treatment with me, which pleased me greatly.

They returned a week later, when he told me he was still sleeping well but would like another shoulder massage because it made him feel so good.

Unfortunately, I was going back to England the next week and wouldn't be back in France for three months. However, his wife was very happy to continue treating him every morning and made an appointment for when I returned.

When they came for this appointment, M. Lesieur walked up to the house almost as quickly as his wife and put his arms around my neck saying "Merci Madame", with tears in his eyes. I quickly said "Please don't thank me – thank your wife!"

He told me he was thrilled because he had been able to do a little bit of painting and was hoping to wallpaper the lounge after another few months.

I saw him again six months later and he was without pain, was sleeping well, walking well, and had even wallpapered their bedroom!

## 10. Spinal – Mining accident

### *Assessment*

Frank had been in a mining accident 19 years previously. A roof beam had fallen on his shoulder, causing serious damage; one of his ribs had been broken and had pierced his lung. Apart from being unable to move his arm away from his side, he was having breathing difficulties, and when walking could only move his feet 15-17 cm at a time. He had been under a consultant for the whole of the 19 years and was becoming progressively worse, rather than better.

His wife had heard me speaking on the radio about the benefits of aromatherapy and decided to try it for Frank. When they arrived, it was obvious that an aromatherapy massage would not be possible – the answer had to be aromaflexology.

His solar plexus, spine, shoulder and lung reflexes on each foot were extremely sensitive, as was the outside of his foot both above and on the elbow reflex. I was hopeful that aromaflexology would help him, even if it took many months.

### *Treatment*

The oils I selected for him, in 30 ml of bland reflex cream base, were:

- black pepper [*Piper nigrum*] – analgesic, antispasmodic
- juniper branch [*Juniperus communis ram.*] – analgesic, antiinflammatory, neurotonic
- frankincense [*Boswellia carteri*] – analgesic, antiinflammatory, cicatrizant, immunostimulant
- lavender [*Lavandula angustifolia*] – analgesic, antispasmodic, calming, general tonic

I gave Frank a treatment twice during the first week, on his solar plexus, neck, shoulder, and lung reflexes, finishing with the kidney reflex. Straight after his first treatment I taught his wife how to work on the reflexes, emphasising the importance of doing it every day – always starting with the solar plexus and finishing with the kidney, ureter and bladder. I was amazed at how quickly she picked it up.

They returned four days later for me to check that she was doing everything correctly – which she was, and doing it very well!

They then came once a week for a further two weeks; once a fortnight for the next month, then once a month. Frank's wife was doing such a good daily job on Frank's feet that eventually they only needed to come once every 2 months. (As I was often teaching abroad, Debbie Moore, a therapist who worked for us, carried out his treatments whilst I was away.)

### *Outcome*

After six weeks it was obvious that Frank's wife had never missed a day, as he could raise his right arm about 10 cm; after another 2 months this had not only increased to 30 cm, but his shoulders and head were half way to being erect and his feet were able to take steps of around 26-30 cm.

After six months, he was leaving the centre with his head erect and an almost normal, albeit slow, step. On his last visit, a year after his first, he proudly showed me how he could now lift his arm almost up to his shoulder and was looking forward to the day he could comb his own hair.

## 11. Spinal – Severe neck problem

### *Assessment*

Edna, a hairdressing client of mine (58), had just recovered from a second hip replacement – on the same hip (the first was not successful) and as the healing of the second one had been helped considerably by aromatherapy, she asked if I could help with the following problem:

She was finding driving difficult as she couldn't easily turn her head and was due to undergo an operation to fuse her cervical vertebrae on account of the severe pain there.

She was very anxious about this, as due to the recent death of her husband she needed to be able to continue driving. She was wearing a surgical collar, which she hated.

I explained that an aromaflexology treatment may be able to help achieve the desired result, and, though she was sceptical about treating the feet to improve movement in her neck, she said she trusted me.

### *Treatment*

She made an appointment and I added the following essential oils to a 30 ml jar of reflex cream base:

- 10 drops rosemary [*Rosmarinus officinalis*] – analgesic, antiinflammatory
- 4 drops sweet marjoram [*Origanum majorana*]– analgesic, antiinflammatory
- 8 drops juniper berry [*Juniperus communis fruct.*] – analgesic, antiinflammatory
- 8 drops lavender [*Lavandula angustifolia*] – analgesic, antiinflammatory

The areas I treated were the solar plexus reflex, her neck reflexes (i.e. all around the base of both big toes), ending with the kidney/bladder reflexes to help expel any toxins. I then showed her how to treat the same areas herself at home every day (with emphasis on every day!) and gave her the jar of reflex cream I had mixed for her.

**Outcome**

At her second visit two weeks later, she told me she had had to go to the doctor's as she had started to have a vaginal discharge. She also said her neck was no better, which both surprised and disappointed me – not even a slight improvement had been made.

During the treatment it turned out that she had been massaging, not around the neck of her big toe, but the soft cushion of the big toe itself, in other words, the pituitary gland reflex, which influences secretions from the sex glands! She had remembered to massage the solar plexus and kidney/bladder reflexes – but – had been massaging the wrong part of her toe! I rectified her mistake (and mine for not giving her a chart!) – and we had a good laugh!

This experience indicated the importance of giving clients a marked chart, showing exactly the position of the reflex points to be massaged, as well as giving the sequence of the treatment.

Happily, 2 weeks later, after treating the correct reflexes, the discharge had stopped and Edna was experiencing less pain and a slight improvement in her neck mobility.

The improvement continued over the next two weeks and at the fourth appointment she arrived smiling – wearing, not the surgical collar she hated, but a collar she had made herself from some foam sponge wrapped in a pretty scarf. She could also now move her neck slightly from side to side without pain.

Six weeks later, with self-treatment daily, plus one by me every two weeks to confirm that all was progressing well, she arrived without even the home-made foam collar – and could turn her neck almost as well as me!

She had just had her last appointment with the consultant prior to the operation and he was so amazed at the improvement in her neck mobility and the lack of pain, that he said the operation would not now be necessary. He also asked her what she had been doing to make such a good recovery – but unfortunately Edna was too embarrassed to say she had been rubbing her big toe!

## 12. Spinal – Whiplash due to accident

**Assessment**

My friend Margaret had been in a car accident and suffered from whiplash as a result. The doctor had simply given her painkillers, saying that it would right itself in time, so she came to the salon to see if there was anything I could do to help.

I suggested an aromaflexology treatment, provided she was prepared to self-treat every day between her visits to me.

### Treatment

I used the same selection of analgesic and antiinflammatory essential oils I had mixed for my trip to Blackpool (Case 6).

I gave her a treatment on her solar plexus, neck and shoulder reflexes, finishing with those of the kidney/bladder, after which I taught her how to do it on herself, giving her the cream I had used and impressing on her how important it was to do it every day. She took her diagram and instructions home and returned four days later for a check, after which she came once more, continuing then to treat herself at home every day.

### Outcome

After a month of daily treatment, Margaret's neck was almost back to normal and when she returned to me for a final check-up, she told me how impressed she was with aromaflexology.

## 13. Stress and Diarrhoea

### Assessment

Mrs. T, 66 years old was suffering from anxiety and frequent diarrhoea. She was experiencing frequent diarrhoea, with occasional stomach cramps.

The reflex assessment confirmed gastrointestinal issues, as well as stress in the solar plexus and neck area.

Another concern was dehydration, as Mrs. T was not drinking much water, nor engaging in her water aerobics, due to her frequent diarrhoea. I recommended that she replace her diet sodas with water, as the former can aggravate diarrhoea, and replace her coffee with roasted chicory or chamomile tea to calm her digestive system.

### Treatment

The following essential oils were added to 30 ml/1 oz. bland cream base :

- 7 drops geranium [*Pelargonium graveolens*] – astringent; decongestant; relaxant
- 5 drops sweet orange [*Citrus aurantium* var. *sinensis* per.] – antispasmodic; calming
- 4 drops sweet marjoram [*Origanum majorana*] – carminative; neurotonic; stomachic
- 4 drops lemon [*Citrus limon*] – antispasmodic; astringent; carminative
- 4 drops ginger [*Zingiber officinale*] carminative; digestive; stomachic
- 3 drops petitgrain [*Citrus aurantium* var. *amara* fol.] – balancing; calming
- 3 drops sandalwood [*Santalum album*] astringent; sedative

After massaging her solar plexus reflex, the neck, digestive and lymph reflexes were treated, finishing with the renal reflexes. Mrs. T was then shown how to massage these herself.

Her instructions were to perform aromaflexology twice daily and to return in one week to check she was doing this correctly.

### Outcome

Two weeks later, Mrs. T reported that the diarrhoea had decreased in frequency, especially during the night. She had also increased her water intake.

She checked with me one month later to report that her diarrhoea had almost completely discontinued. She reported that the regular self-treatments had helped a great deal with both her stress and her diarrhoea.

## 14. Stress with Muscular Tension

### Assessment

On another visit to France, in the north this time, a friend of mine was suffering badly with stress, as her husband had to have a bypass operation. She wasn't sleeping well and her neck ached most of the time.

I gave her a shoulder massage for this, but decided that as I wasn't in France for long I should teach her how to do aromaflexology on herself – on her solar plexus and shoulder reflexes.

### Treatment

The oils selected for Yannick, in 30 ml of bland reflex cream base, were 8 drops each of:

- lemon verbena [*Aloysia triphylla*] – antiinflammatory, calming, sedative, soporific
- Tasmanian blue gum [*Eucalyptus globulus*] – antiinflammatory, rubefacient
- sweet marjoram [*Origanum majorana*]– analgesic, calming, neurotonic
- lavender [*Lavandula officinalis*] – analgesic, antiinflammatory, soporific, general tonic

I treated her solar plexus, neck, shoulder and spinal reflexes, finishing with the kidney/bladder reflexes as usual. I then showed her how to do the treatment on herself (to be done every day!), as her husband was unable to do it for her.

### Outcome

Two weeks later she emailed me to say how much better she was. She kept on with the treatment up to her husband's operation, then for a further month, until he was really on the mend, by which time her stress had naturally subsided.

## 15. Stress, Shoulder Pain and Plantar Fasciitis

### *Assessment*
M Robelet presented with plantar fasciitis, slight stress and muscular pain in her shoulders and mid-lower back. She has been wearing inlays in her trainer-style shoes for 10-12 years (not able to wear other shoes) and suffers from a lot of pain.

### *Treatment*
Essential oils used in 30 ml jar of base cream:

- 10 drops *Zingiber cassamunar* [plai] – antiinflammatory
- 10 drops *Aniba rosaeodora* [rosewood] – analgesic
- 10 drops *Lavandula angustifolia* [lavender] – analgesic, antiinflammatory, calming

### *Outcome*
After her first visit, when she returned one week later, the patient reported that not only did her feet feel much better, but the pain in her shoulders and back had lessened – especially her right shoulder.

On her next visit, one week later, I gave her a warm compress on one foot at a time (using the same essential oils) with a hot hand mitten (popular in France), whilst the other was receiving aromaflexology. The foot was then wrapped in cling film. On her third visit she reported an improvement though not as dramatic as the first time.

At her fourth visit she was generally better; she was finding it easier to walk and had a lot less burning and pain. Her shoulders and back were much the same, but not as bad as when she first came to me.

At her fifth visit two weeks later, she was so much better - with happy feet! She is now keeping to fortnightly visits and once daily self-treatment. She has been shown how to use a compress at home in between visits.

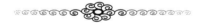

# Chapter Nine
# Essential Oils to Help Health Conditions

There is a specific method of selecting essential oils for an individual client. After completing the assessment, you may find that more than one problem will need help. The following enables the most beneficial essential oils to be selected.

a) Look at the essential oils which are written on the record sheet to help the most important problem (first list)

b) Study those beneficial for the second one. If any of these are in the first list as well, underline them on the first list;

c) Should there be a third problem to help and any of these oils are on your first list, underline them – also on the first list.

By selecting the underlined essential oils you will have a cream which will treat all three problems at the same time. If only one, or two, essential oils is/are repeated, use the majority of drops of these oils, adding the rest from other oils on the first list.

If no oils are repeated, use the greatest number of drops from oils on the first list.

## Essential Oil Choices

- To simplify the listing, only the most frequently used essential oils are mentioned.
- All rosemary [*Rosmarinus officinalis*] cited is the cineole and camphor chemotype.
- All sweet thymes cited below are any of the following chemotypes: *Thymus vulgaris* ct. *geraniol*, ct. *linalool*, ct. *thujanol*-4

## Circulatory system

The circulation is treated automatically during an aromaflexology treatment, whatever the condition being helped, so should the circulation be particularly poor, any circulatory oils appearing in the list of oils in the first column may be underlined in red. If there are none, one or two of the following circulatory oils can be added to column one, the number of drops being used depending on how slow is the circulation:

#### Poor circulation

bitter orange [*Citrus aurantium* var. *amara* per.]; cypress [*Cupressus sempervirens*]; fennel [*Foeniculum vulgare*]; lemon [*Citrus limon*]; rosemary [*Rosmarinus officinalis*]; sage [*Salvia officinalis*]

**Anaemia** (deficiency of red cells or haemoglobin in the blood, resulting in pallor and tiredness).
chamomile Roman [*Chamaemelum nobile*]; lemon [*Citrus limon*]

#### Heart conditions

Before treating clients with the following, permission should be obtained from their GP.
• **Palpitations** (rapid, strong, or irregular heartbeat due to agitation, exertion, or illness)
aniseed [*Pimpinella anisum*]; bitter orange [*Citrus aurantium* var. *amara* per.]; fennel [*Foeniculum vulgare*]; marjoram sweet [*Origanum majorana*]; melissa [*Melissa officinalis*]; peppermint [*Mentha x piperita*]; rosemary [*Rosmarinus officinalis*]; sweet orange [*Citrus sinensis*]
• **Tachycardia** (abnormally rapid heartbeat)
basil [*Ocimum basilicum*]; elecampane [*Inula graveolens*]; lavender [*Lavandula angustifolia*]; lemon verbena [*Aloysia triphylla*]; marjoram sweet [*Origanum majorana*]; ylang ylang [*Cananga odorata*]

#### Hypertension

elecampane [*Inula graveolens*]; lavender [*Lavandula angustifolia*]; lemon [*Citrus limon*]; lemon scented gum [*Eucalyptus citriodora*]; marjoram sweet [*Origanum majorana*]; niaouli [*Melaleuca viridiflora*]; rosemary [*Rosmarinus officinalis*] (low dose); ylang ylang [*Cananga odorata*]

#### Hypotension

basil [*Ocimum basilicum*]; clove bud [*Syzygium aromaticum*]; hyssop [*Hyssopus officinalis*]; peppermint [*Mentha x piperita*]; rosemary [*Rosmarinus officinalis*] (high dose); sage [*Salvia officinalis*]; Scots pine [*Pinus sylvestris*]

## Digestive system

#### Appetite (poor, loss of)

bergamot [*Citrus bergamia*]; caraway [*Carum carvi*]; chamomile Roman [*Chamaemelum nobile*]; fennel [*Foeniculum vulgare*]; ginger [*Zingiber officinale*]; hyssop [*Hyssopus officinalis*]; juniper berry [*Juniperus communis* fruct.]; lemon [*Citrus limon*]; nutmeg [*Myristica fragrans*]; sage [*Salvia officinalis*]; spearmint [*Mentha spicata*]

## Colic
bergamot [*Citrus bergamia*]; cajuput [*Melaleuca leucadendron*]; chamomile Roman [*Chamaemelum nobile*] (intestinal); geranium [*Pelargonium graveolens*]; lavender [*Lavandula angustifolia*]; marjoram sweet [*Origanum majorana*]; peppermint [*Mentha x piperita*]; spearmint [*Mentha spicata*]; ylang ylang [*Cananga odorata*]

## Constipation
bitter orange [*Citrus aurantium* var. *amara* per.]; cornmint [*Mentha arvensis*]; fennel [*Foeniculum vulgare*]; ginger [*Zingiber officinale*]; mandarin [*Citrus reticulata*]; rosemary [*Rosmarinus officinalis*]; spearmint [*Mentha spicata*]; sweet orange [*Citrus sinensis*]

## Diabetes
basil [*Ocimum basilicum*]; geranium [*Pelargonium graveolens*]; juniper berry [*Juniperus communis* fruct.]; lemon [*Citrus limon*]; lemon scented gum [*Eucalyptus citriodora*]; thyme [*Thymus vulgaris* var. sweet]; ylang ylang [*Cananga odorata*]s

## Diarrhoea
clove bud [*Syzygium aromaticum*]; geranium [*Pelargonium graveolens*]; ginger [*Zingiber officinale*]; lemon [*Citrus limon*]; marjoram sweet [*Origanum majorana*]; niaouli [*Melaleuca viridiflora*]; nutmeg [*Myristica fragrans*] (chronic); rosemary [*Rosmarinus officinalis*] (infection); sandalwood [*Santalum album*]; spearmint [*Mentha spicata*]; sweet orange [*Citrus sinensis*] (chronic)

## Infantile diarrhoea
chamomile Roman [*Chamaemelum nobile*]

## Dyspepsia - indigestion
aniseed [*Pimpinella anisum*]; bergamot [*Citrus bergamia*]; bitter orange [*Citrus aurantium* var. *amara* per.]; caraway [*Carum carvi*]; chamomile Roman [*Chamaemelum nobile*]; coriander (*Coriandrum sativum*); cornmint [*Mentha arvensis*]; fennel [*Foeniculum vulgare*]; hyssop [*Hyssopus officinalis*]; mandarin [*Citrus reticulata*]; marjoram sweet [*Origanum majorana*]; peppermint [*Mentha x piperita*]; rosemary [*Rosmarinus officinalis*]; sage [*Salvia officinalis*]; spearmint [*Mentha spicata*]; sweet orange [*Citrus sinensis*]

## Flatulence
basil [*Ocimum basilicum*]; caraway [*Carum carvi*]; chamomile Roman [*Chamaemelum nobile*]; clove bud [*Syzygium aromaticum*]; coriander [*Coriandrum sativum*]; fennel [*Foeniculum vulgare*]; ginger [*Zingiber officinale*]; lavender [*Lavandula angustifolia*]; lemon [*Citrus limon*]; marjoram sweet [*Origanum majorana*]; myrrh [*Commiphora myrrha*]; nutmeg [*Myristica fragrans*]; peppermint [*Mentha x piperita*]; rosemary [*Rosmarinus officinalis*]; spearmint [*Mentha spicata*]

### Gastroenteritis/gastritis

basil [*Ocimum basilicum*]; clove bud [*Syzygium aromaticum*]; coriander [*Coriandrum sativum*]; fennel [*Foeniculum vulgare*]; geranium [*Pelargonium graveolens*]; lemon [*Citrus limon*]; marjoram sweet [*Origanum majorana*]; niaouli [*Melaleuca viridiflora*] (viral); palmarosa [*Cymbopogon martinii*]; patchouli [*Pogostemon patchouli*]; peppermint [*Mentha x piperita*]; ravensara [*Ravensara aromatica*] (viral); rosemary [*Rosmarinus officinalis*]; sage [*Salvia officinalis*] (viral); tea tree [*Melaleuca alternifolia*] (viral)

### Gall bladder malfunction

elecampane [*Inula graveolens*]; Moroccan thyme [*Thymus satureioides*]; rosemary [*Rosmarinus officinalis*] (also for inflamed gall bladder)

### Gall stones

lemon [*Citrus limon*]; niaouli [*Melaleuca viridiflora*]; rosemary [*Rosmarinus officinalis*]; Scots pine [*Pinus sylvestris*]

### Irritable bowel syndrome

black pepper [*Piper nigrum*]; peppermint [*Mentha x piperita*]; sage [*Salvia officinalis*]

### Liver

• **Cirrhosis**

juniper berry [*Juniperus communis* fruct.]; peppermint [*Mentha x piperita*]; rosemary [*Rosmarinus officinalis*]; sage [*Salvia officinalis*]

• **Congestion**

grapefruit [*Citrus paradisi*]; vetiver [*Vetiveria zizanioides*]

• **Inflammation/hepatitis**

basil [*Ocimum basilicum*] (viral); clove bud [*Syzygium aromaticum*]; niaouli [*Melaleuca viridiflora*] (viral); peppermint [*Mentha x piperita*]; ravensara [*Ravensara aromatica*] (viral); rosemary [*Rosmarinus officinalis*];

• **Sluggish**

basil [*Ocimum basilicum*]; black pepper [*Piper nigrum*]; everlasting [*Helichrysum angustifolium*]; geranium [*Pelargonium graveolens*]; melissa [*Melissa officinalis*]; Moroccan chamomile [*Ormenis multicaulis*];

### Painful digestion

ginger [*Zingiber officinale*]; lemon [*Citrus limon*]; mandarin [*Citrus reticulata*]; peppermint [*Mentha x piperita*]; rosemary [*Rosmarinus officinalis*]; sage [*Salvia officinalis*]; Scots pine [*Pinus sylvestris*] (gastric)

### Sluggish digestion

basil [*Ocimum basilicum*]; black pepper [*Piper nigrum*]; coriander [*Coriandrum sativum*];

ginger [*Zingiber officinale*]; gully gum [*Eucalyptus smithii*]; hyssop [*Hyssopus officinalis*]; lemongrass [*Cymbopogon citratus*]; nutmeg [*Myristica fragrans*]; rosemary [*Rosmarinus officinalis*]; sage [*Salvia officinalis*]; spearmint [*Mentha spicata*]

### Stomach cramp
basil [*Ocimum basilicum*] (gastric); bitter orange [*Citrus aurantium* var. *amara* per.]; black spruce [*Picea nigra*]; caraway [*Carum carvi*]; chamomile German [*Matricaria recutita*]; clove bud [*Syzygium aromaticum*] (intestinal); mandarin [*Citrus reticulata*]; melissa [*Melissa officinalis*]; peppermint [*Mentha x piperita*]

## Excretory system

### Cystitis
cajuput [*Melaleuca leucadendron*]; clove bud [*Syzygium aromaticum*]; fennel [*Foeniculum vulgare*]; juniper berry [*Juniperus communis* fruct.]; lavender [*Lavandula angustifolia*]; lemon scented gum [*Eucalyptus citriodora*]; palmarosa [*Cymbopogon martinii*]; peppermint [*Mentha x piperita*]; rosemary [*Rosmarinus officinalis*]; sandalwood [*Santalum album*]; Scots pine [*Pinus sylvestris*]; spearmint [*Mentha spicata*]; Tasmanian blue gum [*Eucalyptus globulus*]; thyme [*Thymus vulgaris* var. sweet]

### Kidney stones
fennel [*Foeniculum vulgare*] (urinary); hyssop [*Hyssopus officinalis*] (urinary); juniper berry [*Juniperus communis* fruct.]; juniper twig [*Juniperus communis* ram.] (urinary); lemon verbena [*Aloysia triphylla*]; sandalwood [*Santalum album*]; Tasmanian blue gum [*Eucalyptus globulus*]; yarrow [*Achillea millefolium*]

## Glandular system

### Hyperthyroidism
cumin [*Cuminum cyminum*]; black spruce [*Picea nigra*]; marjoram sweet [*Origanum majorana*]

### Hypothyroidism
myrtle [*Myrtus communis*]

### Lymph congestion
Atlas cedarwood [*Cedrus atlantica*]; geranium [*Pelargonium graveolens*]; myrtle [*Myrtus communis*]; Scots pine [*Pinus sylvestris*]

## Immune system

### Immuno-deficiency

black peppermint [*Eucalyptus radiata*]; clove bud [*Syzygium aromaticum*]; frankincense [*Boswellia carteri*\*]; Moroccan thyme [*Thymus satureioides*]; niaouli [*Melaleuca viridiflora*]; palmarosa [*Cymbopogon martinii*]; patchouli [*Pogostemon patchouli*]; tea tree [*Melaleuca alternifolia*]; thyme [*Thymus vulgaris* var. sweet]

## Muscular system

### Arthritis/rheumatism: (general, i.e. inflammation and muscular pain)

aniseed [*Pimpinella anisum*]; basil [*Ocimum basilicum*]; cajuput [*Melaleuca leucadendron*]; chamomile Roman [*Chamaemelum nobile*]; clove bud [*Syzygium aromaticum*]; coriander [*Coriandrum sativum*]; frankincense [*Boswellia carteri*]; geranium [*Pelargonium graveolens*]; lavender [*Lavandula angustifolia*]; lemon [*Citrus limon*]; lemon scented gum [*Eucalyptus citriodora*]; marjoram sweet [*Origanum majorana*]; niaouli [*Melaleuca viridiflora*]; nutmeg [*Myristica fragrans*]; Scots pine [*Pinus sylvestris*]; Tasmanian blue gum [*Eucalyptus globulus*];

## Nervous system

### Anxiety/Stress

basil [*Ocimum basilicum*]; bergamot [*Citrus bergamia*]; bitter orange [*Citrus aurantium* var. *amara* per.]; geranium [*Pelargonium graveolens*]; lavender [*Lavandula angustifolia*]; marjoram sweet [*Origanum majorana*]; patchouli [*Pogostemon patchouli*]; petitgrain [*Citrus aurantium* var. *amara* fol.]; sweet orange [*Citrus sinensis*]; thyme population [*Thymus vulgaris*]; ylang ylang [*Cananga odorata*]

### Debility

basil [*Ocimum basilicum*]; clove bud [*Syzygium aromaticum*]; coriander [*Coriandrum sativum*]; cypress [*Cupressus sempervirens*]; geranium [*Pelargonium graveolens*]; juniper branch [*Juniperus communis* ram.]; lavender [*Lavandula angustifolia*]; marjoram sweet [*Origanum majorana*]; rosemary [*Rosmarinus officinalis*]; sage [*Salvia officinalis*]; tea tree [*Melaleuca alternifolia*]

---

\*The '*carteri*' in *Boswellia carteri* (frankincense) is spelt '*carterii*' by some authors. However, the following extract is from 'Botanical Latin' – the book used by The Royal Horticultural Society:
"When the name ends in a consonant, the letters ii are added (thus *ramondii* from Raymond), except when the name ends in er, when a single i is added."

### *Depression*
basil [*Ocimum basilicum*]; chamomile Roman [*Chamaemelum nobile*]; frankincense [*Boswellia carteri*]; marjoram sweet [*Origanum majorana*]; niaouli [*Melaleuca viridiflora*] (post-viral); patchouli [*Pogostemon patchouli*]; petitgrain [*Citrus aurantium* var. *amara* fol.]; 'red' thyme [*Thymus vulgaris* ct. *thymol*, ct. *carvacrol*]; spearmint [*Mentha spicata*]; tea tree [*Melaleuca alternifolia*]; thyme population [*Thymus vulgaris*]

### *Headaches*
basil [*Ocimum basilicum*]; chamomile Roman [*Chamaemelum nobile*]; grapefruit [*Citrus paradisi*]; lavandin [*Lavandula x intermedia*] (chronic); lavender [*Lavandula angustifolia*]; lemon [*Citrus limon*]; marjoram sweet [*Origanum majorana*]; peppermint [*Mentha x piperita*]; rosemary [*Rosmarinus officinalis*]; Tasmanian blue gum [*Eucalyptus globulus*] (congestive)

### *Insomnia*
basil [*Ocimum basilicum*] (nervous); bergamot [*Citrus bergamia*]; chamomile Roman [*Chamaemelum nobile*]; juniper berry [*Juniperus communis* fruct.]; lavender [*Lavandula angustifolia*]; lemon [*Citrus limon*]; mandarin [*Citrus reticulata*]; marjoram sweet [*Origanum majorana*]; sweet orange [*Citrus sinensis*]; thyme [*Thymus vulgaris* var. sweet]; ylang ylang [*Cananga odorata*]

### *Sciatica*
aniseed [*Pimpinella anisum*]; peppermint [*Mentha x piperita*]; 'red' thyme [*Thymus vulgaris* ct. *thymol*, ct. *carvacrol*]; sandalwood [*Santalum album*]

## Reproductive system

### *Menstruation*
• **Amenorrhoea** (abnormal absence)
aniseed [*Pimpinella anisum*]; chamomile Roman [*Chamaemelum nobile*]; clary [*Salvia sclarea*]; niaouli [*Melaleuca viridiflora*]; rosemary [*Rosmarinus officinalis*]; sage [*Salvia officinalis*]
• **Dysmenorrhoea** (painful)
aniseed [*Pimpinella anisum*]; chamomile Roman [*Chamaemelum nobile*]; clary [*Salvia sclarea*]; fennel [*Foeniculum vulgare*]; geranium [*Pelargonium graveolens*]; sage [*Salvia officinalis*]
• **Irregular**
peppermint [*Mentha x piperita*]; sage [*Salvia officinalis*]

### Menopause

aniseed [*Pimpinella anisum*]; chamomile Roman [*Chamaemelum nobile*]; clary [*Salvia sclarea*]; fennel [*Foeniculum vulgare*]; sage [*Salvia officinalis*]

### Oligomenorrhoea (infrequent or scanty)

aniseed [*Pimpinella anisum*]; clary [*Salvia sclarea*]; fennel [*Foeniculum vulgare*]; lavender [*Lavandula angustifolia*]; niaouli [*Melaleuca viridiflora*]; rosemary [*Rosmarinus officinalis*]; sage [*Salvia officinalis*]

### Pre-Menstrual Stress/Tension (PMS/T)

aniseed [*Pimpinella anisum*]; clary [*Salvia sclarea*]; fennel [*Foeniculum vulgare*]; tea tree [*Melaleuca alternifolia*]

### Morning sickness

cardamom [*Elettaria cardamomum*]; lemon [*Citrus limon*]; melissa [*Melissa officinalis*]; peppermint [*Mentha* x *piperita*]; spearmint [*Mentha spicata*]; sweet orange [*Citrus aurantium* var. *sinensis*]

### Ovary problems

cypress [*Cupressus sempervirens*]; fennel [*Foeniculum vulgare*]; myrtle [*Myrtus communis*]; sage [*Salvia officinalis*]

## Respiratory system

### Asthma

aniseed [*Pimpinella anisum*]; frankincense [*Boswellia carteri*]; gully gum [*Eucalyptus smithii*]; hyssop [*Hyssopus officinalis*]; peppermint [*Mentha x piperita*]; sage [*Salvia officinalis*]; Scots pine [*Pinus sylvestris*]; Tasmanian blue gum [*Eucalyptus globulus*]

### Bronchitis

aniseed [*Pimpinella anisum*]; Atlas cedarwood [*Cedrus atlantica*]; black pepper [*Piper nigrum*] (chronic); cajuput [*Melaleuca leucadendron*]; caraway [*Carum carvi*]; cypress [*Cupressus sempervirens*]; frankincense [*Boswellia carteri*]; ginger [*Zingiber officinale*] (chronic); gully gum [*Eucalyptus smithii*]; hyssop [*Hyssopus officinalis*]; juniper twig [*Juniperus communis* ram.]; lavandin [*Lavandula x intermedia*]; marjoram sweet [*Origanum majorana*]; niaouli [*Melaleuca viridiflora*]; peppermint [*Mentha x piperita*]; ravensara [*Ravensara aromatica*]; rosemary [*Rosmarinus officinalis*] (chronic); sage [*Salvia officinalis*]; sandalwood [*Santalum album*] (chronic); Scots pine [*Pinus sylvestris*]; Tasmanian blue gum [*Eucalyptus globulus*] (acute); tea tree [*Melaleuca alternifolia*]; thyme [*Thymus vulgaris* var. sweet]

### Sinusitis

clove bud [*Syzygium aromaticum*]; cornmint [*Mentha arvensis*]; hyssop [*Hyssopus officinalis*]; lavender [*Lavandula angustifolia*]; marjoram sweet [*Origanum majorana*]; myrtle [*Myrtus communis*]; niaouli [*Melaleuca viridiflora*]; peppermint [*Mentha x piperita*]; ravensara [*Ravensara aromatica*]; rosemary [*Rosmarinus officinalis*]; sage [*Salvia officinalis*]; Scots pine [*Pinus sylvestris*]; Tasmanian blue gum [*Eucalyptus globulus*]; thyme [*Thymus vulgaris* var. sweet]

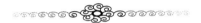

Aromaflexology

# Index

Notes